DR. B. O'NEILL CURE FOR CANCER

Discover Barbara O'Neill's Natural Cancer Treatment: Holistic Healing, Herbal Remedies, and Anti-Cancer Diets for Effective Cancer Prevention and Recovery

DR. LUKA ANDERSON

COPYRIGHT © 2024 BY DR. LUKA ANDERSON

All rights reserved. No part of this publication may be reproduced, distributed, or transmitted in any form or by any means, including photocopying, recording, or other electronic or mechanical methods, without the prior written permission of the publisher, except in the case of brief quotations embodied in critical reviews and certain other noncommercial uses permitted by copyright law.

☐

CHAPTER ONE 7

INTRODUCTION TO NATURAL HEALING AND CANCER PREVENTION 7

Barbara O'Neill's Thoughts 7

REASONS FOR CANCER 10

CANCER TYPES 10

Stages of Cancer 11

CONVENTIONAL VS. NATURAL TREATMENTS 12

Natural Remedies 12

THE VALUE OF MODIFYING ONE'S LIFESTYLE 13

ADVANTAGES OF MODIFYING YOUR LIFESTYLE 14

The Healing Mind-Body Connection 15

Methods to Strengthen the Mind-Body Bond 15

Advantages of Mind-Body Methods 16

CREATING PRACTICAL HEALTH OBJECTIVES 16

How to Make Sense of Your Health Objectives 16

Tracking Development and Modifying Objectives 18

CHAPTER TWO 20

FOODS THAT FIGHT CANCER: NATURE'S PHARMACY 20

Summary of Foods that Fight Cancer 20

Mechanisms of Action 21

THE PHYTOCHEMICALS 22

ANTIOXIDANTS 23

Important Antioxidants 23

FRUITS AND VEGETABLES THAT CAN FIGHT CANCER 24

Cruciferous Produce 24

Berries 25

Fruits of the Citrus 25

Additional Vegetables 26

Whole Grains 26

Legumes 27

INCLUDING NUTS AND SEEDS IN YOUR NUTRITION 28

CHAPTER THREE 31

SUPERFOODS TO ACHIEVE IDEAL HEALTH 31

Specifications of Superfoods... 31

ADVANTAGES OF SUPERFOODS FOR HEALTH........................ 32

The Health Benefits of Leafy Green Vegetables........................ 33

Illustrations of Leafy Green Vegetables 34

GINGER AND TURMERIC: STRONG ANTI-INFLAMMATORIES 36

Turmeric 36

Ginger 37

Garlic 38

Onions 39

THE SEA VEGETABLE'S POWER... 40

SUPERFOOD JUICES AND SMOOTHIES 43

ESSENTIAL COMPONENTS OF SUPERFOOD JUICES AND SMOOTHIES... 44

CHAPTER FOUR 47

ANTI-INFLAMMATORY DIET FOR CANCER PREVENTION 47

Understanding Inflammation and Cancer................................... 47

KEY PRINCIPLES OF AN ANTI-INFLAMMATORY DIET 49

FOODS TO INCLUDE FOR REDUCING INFLAMMATION 50

FOODS TO AVOID FOR BETTER HEALTH 53

Breakfast 54

Lunch 54

Dinner 55

Turmeric Ginger Smoothie 55

Baked Salmon with Lemon and Dill 56

Quinoa and Black Bean Salad 57

Turmeric and Ginger Chicken Soup 58

   TIPS FOR MAINTAINING AN ANTI-INFLAMMATORY LIFESTYLE .. 59

CHAPTER FIVE 61

  ALKALINE DIET: BALANCING YOUR BODY'S PH 61

    The Alkaline Diet: The Science Behind It 61

    THE THEORY OF ACID-ALKALINE 62

    How to Make Alkaline Meals: A Guide and Some Advice 65

    Sample Daily Meal Plans 67

    Monitoring and Adjusting Your pH Balance 72

CHAPTER SIX 76

  KETO-DIETARY APPROACHES TO CANCER TREATMENT 76

    How Cancer Is Fought by Ketosis 77

    Low-Carb, High-Fat Foods to Incorporate 79

    Meal Planning for Keto Dieters 80

    Sample Ketogenic Meal Plans and Recipes 82

    Managing Side Effects of the Ketogenic Diet 85

    Long-Term Advantages and Things to Think About 88

CHAPTER SEVEN 91

  CONSUMING A PLANT-BASED DIET: FUELING YOUR BODY 91

    Vital Elements in Plant-Based Diets 93

- Vegetarian Sources of Protein 94
- Making Plant-Based Meals That Are Balanced 97
- Delicious Plant-Based Recipes 99
- Overcoming Common Challenges.. 102
- Success Stories of People Who Eat Only Plants 105

CHAPTER EIGHT 107
- DETOXIFICATION: SYSTEM PURIFICATION 107
  - The Role of Detoxification in the Healing Process 107
  - Natural Remedy Foods and Beverages 109
  - Safe and Practical Detox Techniques 112
  - Sample Detox Plans and Schedules....................................... 114
  - 7-Day Plant-Based Detox Plan:... 116
  - Recipes for Detoxifying Meals and Smoothies....................... 120
  - Supporting Detox with Lifestyle Changes 127
  - Tracking the Progress of Your Detox...................................... 129

CHAPTER NINE 132
- BOOSTING YOUR IMMUNE SYSTEM ORGANICALLY................. 132

CHAPTER ONE
INTRODUCTION TO NATURAL HEALING AND CANCER PREVENTION

The domains of natural healing and cancer prevention are related to one another and center on the application of holistic, non-invasive techniques to improve general health and stop the growth of cancer. This method combines a number of strategies, including as diet, lifestyle modifications, and mind-body methods, with the goal of strengthening the body's inherent defenses and healing capacities.

Barbara O'Neill's Thoughts

In the fields of holistic health and natural treatment, Barbara O'Neill is well-known. Her concept is based on the idea that, under the correct circumstances, the body has the inherent capacity to heal itself. O'Neill stresses the value of leading a natural lifestyle, which involves eating a healthy diet, detoxifying the body, and getting rid of dangerous drugs.

O'Neill takes a multifaceted approach to health and healing.

1. Nutrition: The importance of nutrition is fundamental to her ideology. She promotes a diet high in unprocessed, whole foods, with a focus on whole grains, fruits, vegetables, nuts, and seeds.

According to her, these foods offer the vital nutrients required for the body to mend itself and perform at its best.

2. Detoxification: O'Neill emphasizes the significance of ridding the body of noxious materials like chemicals, toxins, and processed meals. She frequently suggests doing natural detoxifications using foods that improve liver function, drinking lots of water, and fasting.

3. Lifestyle Modifications: In O'Neill's opinion, lifestyle decisions are crucial to both health and recovery. This include getting enough sleep, exercising frequently, and properly handling stress.

4. Hydrotherapy: O'Neill is a fervent supporter of this pain-relieving and therapeutic method that uses water. According to her, using water treatments can strengthen the immune system, increase blood flow, and aid in the healing process.

5. Herbal medicines: In order to aid the body's healing processes, she also uses herbal medicines. Herbs with anti-inflammatory and antioxidant qualities, such garlic, ginger, and turmeric, can aid in the prevention and treatment of a number of illnesses.

The Function of Diet in Healing and Health

When it comes to preserving health and promoting the body's healing processes, nutrition is essential. Every cell, tissue, and organ in the body is made up of the building blocks found in food. Enough nourishment guarantees that the immune system can successfully combat threats and that the body's systems operate as intended.

Key Nutritional Components

1. Macronutrients: These consist of lipids, proteins, and carbs. Every one has a distinct purpose:

- Energy comes from carbs.
- Tissue upkeep, development, and repair depend on proteins.
- Cell structure, energy storage, and hormone production all depend on fats.

2. Micronutrients: Minerals and vitamins are essential for a number of biological reactions. For example, the immune system benefits from vitamin C, while bone health requires calcium.

3. Phytochemicals: These are substances that are present in plants and have the ability to prevent and treat disease. Examples of substances with anti-inflammatory and antioxidant properties are polyphenols, carotenoids, and flavonoids.

Diet's Effect on Cancer Prevention

It has been demonstrated that a diet high in fruits, vegetables, and whole grains and well-balanced lowers the risk of cancer. These foods are rich in antioxidants, fiber, vitamins, and minerals that can shield cells from oxidative damage that could cause cancer. Particular food suggestions for preventing cancer consist of:

• High Intake of Fiber: Fiber promotes good digestion and aids in the body's removal of impurities.

• Rich in Antioxidants Foods: Free radicals are harmful to cells and can result in cancer. Antioxidants counteract this threat. Nuts, berries, and leafy green vegetables are great sources.

- Good Fats: Omega-3 fatty acids, which can be found in walnuts, flaxseeds, and seafood, have anti-inflammatory qualities that may lower the risk of cancer.

Fundamentals of Cancer: Types, Stages, and Causes

A set of illnesses collectively known as cancer are defined by the unchecked division and proliferation of aberrant cells. Death may ensue if the spread is not stopped.

REASONS FOR CANCER

1. Genetic Elements Hereditary genetic mutations have been connected to certain malignancies. For example, the risk of ovarian and breast cancers is increased by mutations in the BRCA1 and BRCA2 genes.

2. Environmental Factors: The risk of cancer can be raised by exposure to specific chemicals, pollutants, and radiation. For instance, it is commonly recognized that smoking causes lung cancer.

3. Lifestyle Factors: A person's diet, level of physical exercise, and behaviors like drinking and smoking have a big influence on their chance of developing cancer. Numerous cancers have been related to obesity and inactivity.

4. Infections: A number of bacteria and viruses have been linked to cancer. Cervical cancer is associated with the human papillomavirus (HPV), whereas stomach cancer is associated with Helicobacter pylori infection.

CANCER TYPES

Cancer may appear anywhere on the body. Typical varieties include some of the following:

- Carcinomas: These are malignancies of the skin, lungs, breast, and colon that are caused by epithelial cells.

- Sarcomas: These start in the connective tissues, which include cartilage, muscle, and bone.

- Leukemias: These are bone marrow and blood malignancies.

- Lymphomas: These have an impact on the immune system's lymphatic system.

Stages of Cancer

Cancer staging describes the extent of cancer's spread in the body. The most common staging system is the TNM system:

- T (Tumor): Indicates the size and extent of the primary tumor.

- N (Nodes): Describes whether the cancer has spread to nearby lymph nodes.

- M (Metastasis): Indicates whether the cancer has spread to other parts of the body.

Stages are typically grouped into four categories:

- Stage 0: Cancer is in situ, meaning it has not spread.
- Stage I: Cancer is small and localized.

- Stage II: Cancer is larger or has spread to nearby tissues.
- Stage III: Cancer has spread to regional lymph nodes.
- Stage IV: Cancer has spread to distant parts of the body.

CONVENTIONAL VS. NATURAL TREATMENTS

Cancer treatment typically involves a combination of conventional and natural methods. Each approach has its strengths and limitations.

Conventional Treatments

1.Surgery: If the tumor is localized, removing the malignant tissue is frequently the initial step in treatment.

2.Radiation therapy: This modality damages or eliminates cancer cells by using high-energy particles or waves. It can be applied either on its own or in conjunction with other therapies.

3.Chemotherapy: Drugs used to either eradicate or inhibit the growth of cancer cells. Chemotherapy can have adverse effects on healthy and malignant cells.

4.Immunotherapy: This medical intervention strengthens the body's defenses against cancer. It entails the use of chemicals produced in a lab or by the body to enhance or repair immune system performance.

5.Targeted therapy: A medication or combination of substances that specifically targets and destroys cancer cells, usually with minimal harm to healthy cells.

Natural Remedies

Supporting the body's natural healing processes while reducing adverse effects are the main goals of natural remedies. These can be incorporated into a comprehensive cancer care plan or utilized in addition to traditional therapies.

1.Nutrition and Diet: Stressing the benefits of a plant-based diet high in anti-inflammatory and antioxidant foods can help the body heal throughout therapy.

2.Herbal Medicine: There are certain herbs with anti-cancer qualities. Curcumin, for instance, is found in turmeric and has been demonstrated to stop the formation of cancer cells.

3.Acupuncture: Helps reduce adverse effects from traditional therapies, like fatigue and nausea, and assist control pain.

4.Mind-Body Therapies: Methods like yoga, meditation, and guided imagery help boost immunity, lessen stress, and enhance overall quality of life.

5.Exercise: Getting regular exercise can boost mood, lessen weariness, and improve general health.

THE VALUE OF MODIFYING ONE'S LIFESTYLE

Modifications in lifestyle are crucial for cancer prevention as well as for promoting healing during and after treatment. The general health and well-being may be significantly impacted by these modifications.

Important Lifestyle Adjustments

1. A healthy diet that emphasizes whole foods, such as an abundance of fruits and vegetables, can lower the risk of cancer and enhance general health.

2. Frequent Exercise: Exercise strengthens the immune system, lowers inflammation, and aids in maintaining a healthy weight. Try to get in at least 150 minutes a week of moderate activity.

3. Steer clear of Tobacco and Excessive Alcohol: Smoking is one of the main causes of cancer, and drinking too much alcohol has been connected to a number of cancers, including liver, breast, and colon cancer.

4. Sufficient Sleep: Immune system performance and general health depend on getting enough good sleep. 7 to 9 hours each night is the goal.

5. Stress management: Prolonged stress can impair immunity and increase the risk of developing cancer. Stress management techniques include deep breathing, mindfulness, and meditation.

ADVANTAGES OF MODIFYING YOUR LIFESTYLE

- Enhanced Immune Function: Living a healthy lifestyle helps the immune system function better, which increases its capacity to identify and eliminate cancer cells.

- Decreased Inflammation: Inflammation is a common symptom of many chronic illnesses, including cancer. Inflammation can be decreased with anti-inflammatory diets and frequent exercise.

- Better Mental Health: Stress reduction and physical exercise lift the spirits and lessen anxiety and depression, which are prevalent in cancer patients.

The Healing Mind-Body Connection

The tremendous impact that mental and emotional states have on physical health is known as the "mind-body connection." This relationship is especially significant for cancer patients since stress, worry, and depression can have a deleterious effect on immune system performance and general health.

Methods to Strengthen the Mind-Body Bond

1.Meditation: Consistent meditation practice lowers blood pressure, eases stress, and enhances emotional health. In particular, mindfulness meditation facilitates stress management and present-moment awareness.

2.Yoga: Blends meditation, breathing techniques, and physical postures. Yoga can increase mental clarity, decrease stress, and increase flexibility.

3.Using guided imagery, one can picture healing and beneficial results. This method can ease tension, encourage calmness, and elevate mood.

4.Biofeedback: teaches people how to regulate physiological processes like heart rate and muscular tension using electronic instruments. Stress and pain can be effectively managed using biofeedback.

5.Psychotherapy: Patients can manage the psychological effects of cancer with the assistance of counseling and therapy. Positive behavioral improvements and the addressing of negative thought patterns are particularly well-served by cognitive-behavioral therapy, or CBT.

Advantages of Mind-Body Methods

• Less Stress: Immune system performance and general health can both benefit from less stress.

• Better Quality of Life: Mind-body practitioners frequently claim more emotional stability and a higher quality of life.

• Improved Treatment Outcomes: Reducing stress and maintaining a positive outlook can make traditional cancer therapies more successful.

CREATING PRACTICAL HEALTH OBJECTIVES

In order to stay motivated and achieve long-term success in cancer prevention and treatment, it is imperative to set realistic health objectives. Objectives ought to be time-bound, relevant, measurable, achievable, and specific (SMART).

How to Make Sense of Your Health Objectives

1. Assess existing Health: To start, assess your existing state of health, taking a look at your stress levels, sleep patterns, nutrition, and physical activity. Determine which locations require development.

2.Establish Clear and Specific Goals: Establish precise goals. Specify your aim to be "eat at least five servings of fruits and vegetables daily" rather than just "eat healthier."

3.Make Your Goals Measurable: Make sure your objectives are quantifiable. If your objective is to exercise more, for instance, choose how many hours or minutes you will dedicate to physical activity each week.

4.Make Sure Your Goals Can Be Attained: Make sure your goals are difficult but doable. If you don't already exercise, try starting off with 10 minutes a day and working your way up.

5.Relevance is Key: Ensure that your objectives are pertinent to both your general well-being and cancer prevention plan. Every target should support your long-term health goals.

6.Time-Bound Objectives: Establish a timeframe for accomplishing your objectives. This keeps things in perspective and gives off a sense of urgency. For example, set a goal to lose a specific amount of weight in six months.

Realistic Health Goal Examples

- Dietary Modifications: "At least five times a week, swap out sugary snacks for fresh fruit."

- Exercise: "Walk for thirty minutes, five days a week."

- Stress Reduction: "Each morning, spend ten minutes practicing mindfulness meditation."

"Establish a bedtime routine to get at least 7 hours of sleep each night." is the recommendation for improving sleep.

Tracking Development and Modifying Objectives

Track your advancement toward your health objectives on a regular basis. Use a smartphone app or a journal to record your successes and setbacks. If you hit a roadblock, evaluate the situation and modify your objectives accordingly. Being adaptable is crucial; mistakes should not be seen as failures but rather as chances to grow and change.

Looking for Assistance

Having other people's support makes achieving health goals frequently easier. Tell those you want to reach your goals—friends, family, or a medical professional—so they can support and hold you accountable. Insight and direction can also be obtained by joining communities or support groups centered around health. An all-encompassing approach to health that include diet, lifestyle modifications, and mind-body practices is what is meant by natural healing and cancer prevention. The philosophy of Barbara O'Neill emphasizes how the body has the inherent capacity to cure itself with the help of a good diet, cleansing, and way of living. For the sake of prevention and therapy, it is essential to comprehend the fundamentals of cancer, including its forms, causes, and stages. In the treatment of cancer, both conventional and alternative therapies have their place, and combining the two can improve results overall. A good diet, frequent exercise, and stress reduction are examples of lifestyle modifications that are essential for both preventing cancer and promoting recovery. Healing is greatly influenced by the mind-body link, with practices like yoga and meditation enhancing both mental and physical well-being. Achieving long-term health and well-being requires regular progress monitoring and setting realistic health objectives. A holistic approach to health can greatly lower a person's risk of cancer and improve their quality of life in general.

CHAPTER TWO
FOODS THAT FIGHT CANCER: NATURE'S PHARMACY

The theory behind anticancer foods is that some foods have ingredients that can stop, slow down, or even stop the formation of malignant cells. Such foods are abundant in nature and are bursting with potent nutrients, phytochemicals, and antioxidants that promote general well-being and strengthen the body's defenses against cancer. This in-depth manual explores the world of anticancer foods, their qualities, and how they support general health and cancer prevention.

Summary of Foods that Fight Cancer

Generally plant-based, anticancer foods are renowned for their abundance in vitamins, minerals, antioxidants, and phytochemicals. These meals can strengthen the immune system, lower inflammation, and shield cells from harm, increasing the body's ability to fight cancerous cells. The strongest anticancer foods are whole grains, legumes, nuts, seeds, fruits, and vegetables.

Diet's Significance in Cancer Prevention

A key component of cancer prevention is diet. Research indicates that between 30 and 40 percent of cancer cases are thought to be related to dietary variables. Eating a diet high in plant-based foods can dramatically reduce the incidence of prostate, colon, and breast cancer, among other cancers. In addition to offering vital nutrients, these meals comprise ingredients that have been demonstrated to impede the growth and spread of cancer cells.

Mechanisms of Action

Foods anticancer agents function via multiple mechanisms:

• Antioxidant Activity: Free radicals are unstable chemicals that can harm DNA and other biological components, ultimately resulting in cancer. Antioxidants neutralize free radicals.

• Anti-Inflammatory Properties: A higher risk of cancer has been associated with chronic inflammation. The anti-inflammatory properties of several anticancer foods can aid in lowering this risk.

• Detoxification: Certain meals aid in the body's removal of toxins and other dangerous chemicals by supporting its detoxification processes.

• Hormonal Balance: Certain meals can affect metabolism and hormone levels, which lowers the risk of diseases linked to hormones, such as prostate and breast cancer.

• Immune Support: By strengthening immune system performance, anticancer foods help the body recognize and eliminate cancer cells more successfully.

An explanation of phytochemicals and antioxidants

The main ingredients that give anticancer foods their potent health effects are phytochemicals and antioxidants. Comprehending these substances and their mechanisms of action can help explain why specific diets are so successful in avoiding cancer.

THE PHYTOCHEMICALS

Plants naturally contain substances called phytochemicals. They provide major health benefits, especially in preventing and combating cancer, although they are not necessary nutrients like vitamins and minerals. Phytochemicals come in thousands of varieties, and each has special qualities.

Phytochemical Types

1.Flavonoids: Rich in antioxidants and anti-inflammatory qualities, flavonoids can be found in fruits, vegetables, tea, and wine. Quercetin (found in apples and onions) and catechins (found in green tea) are two examples.

2.Carotenoids are pigments that are responsible for the vivid hues of fruits and vegetables. These include lutein (found in leafy greens), lycopene (found in tomatoes), and beta-carotene (found in carrots and sweet potatoes).

3.Glucosinolates: Found in cruciferous vegetables such as Brussels sprouts and broccoli, glucosinolates have the ability to be transformed into physiologically active substances with anticancer qualities.

4.Polyphenols: Rich in antioxidants, these substances are present in foods such as nuts, seeds, and berries. Examples are ellagic acid (found in berries) and resveratrol (found in red wine and grapes).

5.Legumes include saponins, which have been demonstrated to boost the immune system and stop the proliferation of cancer cells.

ANTIOXIDANTS

Molecules called antioxidants shield cells from harm brought on by free radicals. Highly reactive chemicals known as free radicals can induce oxidative stress, which damages cells and raises the risk of cancer. Free radicals are neutralized by antioxidants, averting this harm.

Important Antioxidants

1.Vitamin C: Rich in antioxidants that boost immunity and shield cells from harm, vitamin C is present in citrus fruits, strawberries, and bell peppers.

2.Vitamin E: Rich in leafy greens, nuts, and seeds, vitamin E aids in preventing oxidative damage to cell membranes.

3.Beta-Carotene: An antioxidant that is present in orange and yellow fruits and vegetables, beta-carotene is a precursor to vitamin A.

4.Selenium: Found in whole grains, fish, and Brazil nuts, selenium is a mineral with antioxidant qualities.

5.Polyphenols: Polyphenols have potent antioxidant qualities in addition to the advantages of phytochemicals. Many plant-based foods, such as tea, coffee, and dark chocolate, contain them.

FRUITS AND VEGETABLES THAT CAN FIGHT CANCER

The foundation of any diet designed to prevent cancer is fruits and vegetables. They offer a variety of vitamins, minerals, and phytochemicals that function in concert to prevent cancer.

Cruciferous Produce

Vegetables that are cruciferous are especially powerful anticancer nutrients. Broccoli, cauliflower, Brussels sprouts, kale, and cabbage are some of them. Glucosinolates, sulfur-containing chemicals that can be transformed into biologically active molecules like isothiocyanates and indoles, are abundant in these vegetables. Through their ability to detoxify carcinogens, shield cells from DNA damage, and cause cancer cells to undergo apoptosis (programmed cell death), these chemicals have been demonstrated to impede the development of cancer.

Particular Advantages

1.Broccoli: HDAC, an enzyme involved in the growth of cancer, is inhibited by sulforaphane, which has been demonstrated to have anticancer benefits via increasing phase II detoxifying enzymes.

2.Kale: Packed with glucosinolates, vitamins C and K, and antioxidants. It has been demonstrated that kale lowers the risk of prostate, ovarian, breast, colon, and bladder cancers.

3.Brussels sprouts: Packed with antioxidants and glucosinolates, Brussels sprouts have been demonstrated to guard against DNA damage and lower the risk of a number of cancer types.

Berries

Some of the most potent anticancer foods are berries, including blueberries, strawberries, raspberries, and blackberries. They are abundant in fiber, vitamins, and polyphenols, such as tannins and flavonoids, which have potent anti-inflammatory and antioxidant qualities.

Particular Advantages

1.High concentrations of anthocyanins, which have been demonstrated to stop cancer cells from growing and to cause apoptosis, are present in blueberries.

2.Strawberries: Packed in vitamin C and ellagic acid, which has been demonstrated to guard against esophageal, lung, bladder, and skin cancers.

3.Raspberries: These berries are rich in antioxidant and anti-inflammatory compounds called quercetin and ellagic acid, which may help prevent cancer.

Fruits of the Citrus

Citrus fruits, such as grapefruits, oranges, lemons, and limes, are high in limonoids, flavonoids, and vitamin C, all of which support their anticancer characteristics.

Particular Advantages

1.Oranges: Rich in vitamin C, which boosts immunity and guards against oxidative damage to DNA.

2.Lemons: Studies have indicated that the limonoids found in lemons cause cancer cells to undergo apoptosis.

3.Grapefruits: Packed in naringenin, a flavonoid that has been demonstrated to stop cancer cells from growing.

Additional Vegetables

1.Tomatoes: Packed with lycopene, a potent antioxidant that has been demonstrated to lower the risk of cancer, including prostate cancer.

2.Beta-carotene, which possesses antioxidant qualities and can shield cells from harm, is present in carrots.

3.Rich in flavonoids, zeaxanthin, and lutein, spinach has been demonstrated to offer protection against a number of cancer types.

Complete Grains & Legumes for Well-Being

Legumes and whole grains are crucial parts of a diet that fights cancer. They offer a wealth of phytochemicals, vitamins, minerals, and fiber that promote general health and lower the risk of cancer.

Whole Grains

Nutrient- and fiber-dense whole grains include brown rice, oats, quinoa, barley, and whole wheat. They undergo very little processing and keep the bran, germ, and endosperm of the grain.

Advantages of Whole Grains

1.Dietary fiber, which is abundant in whole grains, aids in blood sugar regulation, proper digestion, and weight management. Additionally, fiber aids in clearing the digestive tract of carcinogens.

2.Antioxidants: Antioxidants like phenolic acids, vitamin E, and selenium are found in whole grains and help shield cells from harm.

3.Phytochemicals: It has been demonstrated that the presence of phytochemicals like saponins and lignans in whole grains lowers the risk of cancer.

Legumes

Beans, lentils, chickpeas, and peas are examples of legumes that are high in fiber, protein, and minerals. Their anticancer activities are also attributed to the range of phytochemicals they contain.

Advantages of Legume

1.Plant-based protein, found in legumes, is essential for immune system and cell repair.

2.Fiber: A high fiber diet promotes the body's ability to eliminate carcinogens from the body and regulates digestion.

3.Phytochemicals: Research has demonstrated that the saponins, protease inhibitors, and phytates found in legumes can impede the growth of cancer cells and lower the risk of developing the disease.

Particular Plants

1.Black beans: Rich in saponins and anthocyanins, which have been demonstrated to stop the growth of cancer cells.

2.Lentils: Packed with fiber, folate, and polyphenols, which are known to have anti-inflammatory and antioxidant qualities.

3.Chickpeas: Have been demonstrated to possess anticancer properties due to their saponins and protease inhibitors.

INCLUDING NUTS AND SEEDS IN YOUR NUTRITION

Nuts and seeds are foods high in nutrients, including protein, healthy fats, vitamins, minerals, and phytochemicals. They are simple to include in the diet and have been found to offer a host of health advantages, including a potential defense against cancer.

Advantages of Nuts

Nuts high in healthful fats, especially omega-3 and omega-6 fatty acids, include cashews, walnuts, almonds, and Brazil nuts. They also offer fiber, vitamins, minerals, and protein.

Particular Advantages

1. Almonds: Rich in vitamin E, which helps shield cells from harm and has antioxidant qualities.

2. Walnuts: Research has demonstrated that the omega-3 fatty acids and polyphenols found in walnuts help lower inflammation and stop the formation of cancer cells.

3. Extremely high in selenium, a potent antioxidant that boosts immunity and lowers cancer risk, are Brazil nuts.

Advantages of Seeds

Rich in protein, fiber, healthy fats, vitamins, and minerals, seeds including flaxseeds, chia seeds, pumpkin seeds, and sunflower seeds are also a good source of these nutrients.

Particular Advantages

1. Flaxseeds: Rich in lignans and omega-3 fatty acids, which have been demonstrated to lower the incidence of prostate and breast cancer.

2. Chia seeds: Packed in antioxidants, fiber, and omega-3 fatty acids, which promote general well-being and lower inflammation.

3. Pumpkin Seeds: Studies have indicated that the phytosterols and antioxidants in pumpkin seeds promote prostate health and lower the risk of cancer.

How to Include Seeds and Nuts

1. Snacking: A quick and wholesome snack is nuts and seeds. Have a variety of your preferred nuts and seeds on hand for an easy, wholesome snack.

2. Smoothies: To add even more nutrients to your morning smoothie, try adding a tablespoon of hemp, chia, or flaxseeds.

3. Salads: To enhance texture, flavor, and nutritional value, sprinkle nuts or seeds on top of salads.

4. Baking: To boost the nutritional value of baked goods like muffins, breads, and cookies, add nuts and seeds to the mixture.

5. Breakfast: For a wholesome start to the day, add nuts or seeds to your cereal, yogurt, or oatmeal.

Foods high in antioxidants are an effective weapon in the battle against cancer. You may dramatically lower your risk of cancer and improve your general health by learning about the functions of phytochemicals and antioxidants and including a range of fruits, vegetables, whole grains, legumes, nuts, and seeds in your diet. Adopting a varied, plant-based diet full of these nutrient-dense foods is essential since they complement each other's actions to prevent cancer and promote the body's natural healing processes.

CHAPTER THREE
SUPERFOODS TO ACHIEVE IDEAL HEALTH

Superfoods are foods high in nutrients that are thought to be particularly advantageous for overall health and wellbeing. Their abundance of vitamins, minerals, antioxidants, and other nutrients offers a plethora of health advantages, such as heightened energy, less inflammation, better immune system performance, and a decreased chance of chronic illnesses. This in-depth guide explores the realm of superfoods, their advantages, and how to include them in a balanced diet for optimum health.

Superfoods: What Are They?

Superfoods are whole, high-nutrient foods that offer major health advantages over standard diets. Generally speaking, they are abundant in vitamins, minerals, antioxidants, and other bioactive substances that support a variety of body processes and aid in disease prevention. The phrase "superfood" is a marketing word intended to emphasize the better nutritional profile and health advantages of particular foods, not a scientific certification.

Specifications of Superfoods

1. High Nutrient Density: Compared to their calorie count, superfoods have a high concentration of vital nutrients.

2.Antioxidant Rich: They contain a lot of antioxidants, which help prevent oxidative stress and neutralize dangerous free radicals.

3.Anti-Inflammatory Properties: Anti-inflammatory substances found in a lot of superfoods can aid in reducing chronic inflammation, which is a key cause of a number of ailments.

4.Unique bioactive substances found in them have the potential to improve health and fend off disease.

ADVANTAGES OF SUPERFOODS FOR HEALTH

1.Enhanced Immune Function: By strengthening the immune system, superfoods might make it easier for the body to fend against infections and illnesses.

2.Decreased Inflammation: Superfoods' anti-inflammatory qualities can aid in reducing long-term inflammation, which lowers the chance of developing long-term conditions like diabetes, arthritis, and heart disease.

3.Better Digestive Health: High fiber content in superfoods promotes a healthy digestive system and helps ward off constipation.

4.Improved Heart Health: The presence of certain nutrients in superfoods, like fiber, antioxidants, and omega-3 fatty acids, can lower the risk of heart disease and enhance cardiovascular health.

5.Cancer Prevention: It has been demonstrated that certain superfoods include substances that stop the growth of cancer cells and lower the chance of developing different kinds of cancer.

6.Enhanced Vitality and Energy: Superfoods' rich nutritional makeup might assist increase vitality and energy levels in general.

The Health Benefits of Leafy Green Vegetables

Rich in vitamins, minerals, antioxidants, and fiber, green leafy vegetables are among the healthiest foods out there, providing a plethora of health advantages. Arugula, collard greens, spinach, kale, and Swiss chard are a few examples.

Profile of Nutrition

While low in calories, green leafy vegetables are high in vital nutrients, such as:

- **Vitamins:** several B vitamins, A, C, and K.

- **Minerals:** potassium, iron, magnesium, and calcium.

- Zeaxanthin, lutein, and beta-carotene are antioxidants.

- **Fiber:** Fiber, both soluble and insoluble, promotes the health of the digestive system.

Advantages for Health

1.Strong in vitamin K, which is necessary for strong bones and aids in the synthesis of osteocalcin, a protein that attaches calcium to bones.

2.Eye Health: High in antioxidants such as lutein and zeaxanthin, which shield the eyes from damaging light and lower the risk of age-related macular degeneration.

3.Heart Health: Nitrates are present and can help decrease blood pressure and enhance heart health.

4.Digestive Health: The high fiber content helps to avoid constipation and encourages a healthy digestive system.

5.Cancer Prevention: The cruciferous greens (kale, for example) contain compounds called glucosinolates that help detoxify the body and lower the risk of cancer.

Illustrations of Leafy Green Vegetables

1.Rich in iron, magnesium, and folate, spinach promotes the body's ability to produce energy and maintain general health.

2.Kale: Rich in antioxidants and vitamins A, C, and K, kale has potent anti-inflammatory properties.

3.Swiss Chard: A good source of potassium, magnesium, and the vitamins A, C, and K.

4.Nitrates and antioxidants found in arugula help to lower inflammation and promote cardiovascular health.

5.Collard Greens: Rich in vitamin K and calcium, collard greens promote healthy bones and general wellbeing.

The Value of Dark Fruits and Berries

Dark fruits and berries are rich in nutrients and deliciousness. They are abundant in vitamins, fiber, antioxidants, and other bioactive substances that have a host of positive health effects.

Profile of Nutrition

Dark fruits and berries are abundant in:

- Vitamins: calcium and vitamin K in particular.

Magnese, potassium, and magnesium are examples of minerals.

- Antioxidants: polyphenols, flavonoids, and anthocyanins.

- Fiber: Both soluble and insoluble fiber promotes the health of the digestive system.

Advantages for Health

1. Antioxidant Powerhouse: Berries include high quantities of antioxidants that lower the risk of chronic diseases and shield cells from oxidative damage.

2. Anti-Inflammatory Properties: Berries' bioactive ingredients can help lessen inflammation and the chance of developing inflammatory illnesses.

3. Heart Health: Berries help lower blood pressure, improve cholesterol, and lower the risk of heart disease.

4. Cancer Prevention: Studies have demonstrated that berries, specifically ellagic acid, contain chemicals that impede the formation of cancer cells.

5. Cognitive Health: Berries include antioxidants that may help shield the brain from oxidative stress and enhance cognitive performance.

Berries with Dark Fruit Examples

1. Anthocyanins, found in abundance in blueberries, are powerful antioxidants that promote brain function.

2.Strawberries: Rich in flavonoids and vitamin C, strawberries can lower inflammation and strengthen the heart.

3.Raspberries: Have anticancer qualities due to the presence of quercetin and ellagic acid.

4.Blackberries: Rich in fiber, anthocyanins, vitamins C and K, and other nutrients, blackberries boost immunity and general well-being.

5.Cherries: Packed in anti-inflammatory and antioxidant properties, cherries help relieve aches in the muscles and promote heart health.

GINGER AND TURMERIC: STRONG ANTI-INFLAMMATORIES

Spices like ginger and turmeric are well-known for their potent antioxidant and anti-inflammatory qualities. They have been used for millennia to cure a wide range of illnesses and enhance general health in traditional medicine.

Turmeric

The brilliant yellow spice known as turmeric is made from the Curcuma longa plant's root. Many of its health advantages are attributed to curcumin, the molecule that is active in it.

Turmeric's Health Benefits

1.Anti-Inflammatory: A strong anti-inflammatory substance called curcumin can help lessen chronic inflammation and soothe the signs and symptoms of inflammatory illnesses.

2.Strong antioxidant qualities found in curcumin shield cells from oxidative harm.

3.discomfort Relief: For those with osteoarthritis, turmeric can help lessen discomfort and enhance function.

4.Heart Health: Curcumin lowers the risk of heart disease and enhances endothelial function.

5.Brain Health: Curcumin has the ability to raise brain-derived neurotrophic factor (BDNF), which lowers the risk of neurodegenerative illnesses and supports brain function.

6.Cancer Prevention: It has been demonstrated that curcumin inhibits the growth of cancer cells and lowers the chance of developing several kinds of cancer.

Ginger

The Zingiber officinale plant's rhizome is used to make ginger, a spice. Because of its therapeutic qualities, traditional medicine has long used it.

Ginger's Health Benefits

1.Anti-Inflammatory: The potent anti-inflammatory compounds found in ginger are called gingerols and shogaols.

2.Digestive Health: Ginger helps lessen bloating, enhance digestion, and ease nausea.

3.Pain Relief: Ginger helps lessen osteoarthritis symptoms, including soreness and pain in the muscles.

4.Heart Health: Ginger has been shown to lower blood pressure, cholesterol, and enhance cardiovascular health.

5.Strong antioxidant qualities found in ginger help shield cells from oxidative harm.

6.Immune Support: Ginger helps strengthen the body's defenses against illness.

How to Include Ginger and Turmeric

1.Teas: To make a calming and anti-inflammatory beverage, steep ginger and turmeric teas.

2.Smoothies: For an added health benefit, including fresh or powdered ginger and turmeric in your smoothies.

3.Cooking: In curries, soups, and stir-fries, use turmeric and ginger as ingredients.

4.Supplements: If you'd want a concentrated dose of the active ingredients in turmeric and ginger, there are supplements available.

Onions and Garlic: Organic Detoxifiers

As members of the allium family, garlic and onions are renowned for their potent tastes and wide range of health advantages. Sulfur compounds found in them have strong cleansing and health-promoting effects.

Garlic

For thousands of years, people have utilized the medicinal benefits of garlic, a bulbous plant, for various purposes. A large number of its health advantages are attributed to its active ingredient, allicin.

Garlic's Health Benefits

1.Garlic supports liver function and increases the synthesis of detoxifying enzymes, which aid in the body's detoxification process.

2.Immune Support: The antibacterial and immune-stimulating qualities of garlic aid in the prevention of infections.

3.Heart Health: Garlic helps lower blood pressure, cholesterol, and enhance cardiovascular health.

4.Anti-Inflammatory: The anti-inflammatory qualities of garlic may help lower the chance of developing chronic illnesses.

5.Antioxidant: The antioxidants in garlic lessen oxidative stress and shield cells from harm.

6.Cancer Prevention: Studies have demonstrated that some compounds in garlic can stop the spread of cancer cells and lower the incidence of several cancer forms.

Onions

A vegetable with many uses, onions are available in red, yellow, and white hues. They are abundant in minerals, vitamins, and bioactive substances.

Onions' Health Benefits

1.Detoxification: Sulfur-containing chemicals found in onions aid in liver function and improve detoxification procedures.

2.Immune Support: The antibacterial qualities of onions help strengthen the immune system and stave off illnesses.

3.Heart Health: Onions have been shown to lower blood pressure, cholesterol, and enhance cardiovascular health.

4.Anti-Inflammatory: Onions' ability to reduce inflammation may help lower the chance of developing chronic illnesses.

5.Antioxidant: Quercetin, one of the several antioxidants found in onions, helps shield cells from oxidative damage.

6.Cancer Prevention: It has been demonstrated that some compounds in onions stop the growth of cancer cells and lower the chance of developing different kinds of cancer.

How to Include Onions and Garlic

1.Cooking: To make soups, stews, stir-fries, and sauces, start with onions and garlic.

2.Raw: For a powerful health boost, add raw onions and garlic to salads, salsas, and sauces.

3.Roasting: To lend a softer, sweeter flavor to a variety of meals, roast garlic and onions.

4.Supplements: For people who wish to gain the benefits of garlic's active ingredients without eating a lot of the vegetable, supplements are available.

THE SEA VEGETABLE'S POWER

Sea vegetables, sometimes referred to as seaweeds, are a very nutrient-dense but sometimes disregarded class of superfoods. They are abundant in antioxidants, vitamins, minerals, and other bioactive substances that offer a variety of health advantages.

Sea Vegetable Types

1. Nori: A form of red seaweed high in protein, vitamins, and minerals, nori is frequently used in sushi.

2. Brown seaweed known as "kelp" has a high iodine content, which is necessary for thyroid function.

3. Dulse: A red seaweed high in minerals, iron, and protein.

4. Wakame: A vitamin- and mineral-rich brown seaweed that's frequently added to salads and soups.

5. Kombu: A kelp variety rich in iodine and other minerals that is used in soups and broths.

Profile of Nutrition

Because of their extraordinary nutritious density, sea veggies offer:

- Vitamins: several B vitamins, A, C, E, and K.

- Minerals: potassium, iron, calcium, magnesium, and iodine.

- Flavonoids, polyphenols, and fucoxanthin are antioxidants.

- Fiber: Both soluble and insoluble fiber promote healthy digestion.

- Omega-3 Fatty Acids: Vital for heart and brain function.

Advantages for Health

1. Thyroid Health: One of the best organic sources of iodine, which is necessary for the synthesis of thyroid hormones, is sea vegetables.

2.Detoxification: By binding to heavy metals and other pollutants and promoting their removal from the body, sea vegetables can aid in detoxification.

3.Heart Health: Sea veggies' fiber, antioxidants, and omega-3 fatty acids promote heart health by lowering the risk of heart disease.

4.Anti-Inflammatory: The anti-inflammatory chemicals found in sea veggies can help lower inflammation and the chance of developing chronic illnesses.

5.Digestive Health: The high fiber content helps to avoid constipation and encourages a healthy digestive system.

6.Cancer Prevention: Research has demonstrated that certain chemicals in sea veggies can stop the spread of cancer cells and lower the chance of developing different kinds of the disease.

How to Include Maritime Vegetables

1.Sushi: To produce sushi rolls, use nori sheets.

2.Soups: To enhance taste and nutrients, add wakame or kombu to soups and broths.

3.Salads: To add extra nutrients, add wakame or dulse to your salads.

4.Snacks: For a nutrient-dense, healthful snack, try roasted seaweed snacks.

5.Supplements: If you'd like to acquire the nutrients from sea vegetables without eating them, there are supplements available.

SUPERFOOD JUICES AND SMOOTHIES

You can get a range of nutrient-dense foods into your diet by making superfood juices and smoothies. They can be customized to match your unique health needs and preferences and are quick and easy.

Superfood Juices and Smoothies' Advantages

1.Vitamin Density: A single serving of smoothies and juices can have a high concentration of vitamins, minerals, antioxidants, and other nutrients.

2.Digestibility: Fruits and vegetables' fiber and cell walls are broken down by blending and juicing, which facilitates the body's easier absorption of nutrients.

3.Convenience: Juices and smoothies are an easy method to improve your consumption of superfoods because they're portable and easy to make.

4.Customizable: Depending on your dietary requirements and taste preferences, you can add a range of superfoods to smoothies and juices.

ESSENTIAL COMPONENTS OF SUPERFOOD JUICES AND SMOOTHIES

1.Leafy Greens: When added to smoothies and juices, leafy greens like spinach, kale, Swiss chard, and others provide vitamins, minerals, and fiber.

2.Berries & Fruits: A variety of nutrients and natural sweetness are added by apples, bananas, strawberries, raspberries, and blueberries.

3.Nut butters, avocado, chia seeds, and flaxseeds are good sources of healthy fats that enhance nutrient absorption.

4.Protein: To help keep you full and maintain muscular health, add protein to your diet with Greek yogurt, protein powder, or nut butters.

5.Superfood Powders: To add even more nutrients, mix in powders like acai, maca, spirulina, or chlorella.

6.Spices: Ginger, cinnamon, and turmeric enhance flavor and have anti-inflammatory properties.

Recipes for Superfood Smoothies

1.Smoothie: Combine spinach, kale, cucumber, apple, lemon juice, and chia seeds with a tablespoon for a revitalizing and cleansing smoothie.

2.Berry Blast Smoothie: For an antioxidant-rich smoothie, blend together mixed berries (strawberries, raspberries, and blueberries), Greek yogurt, banana, and a tablespoon of flaxseed.

3.Tropical Turmeric Smoothie: For an anti-inflammatory smoothie, blend together mango, pineapple, banana, coconut water, a teaspoon of turmeric, and a tablespoon of chia seeds.

4.Chocolate Avocado Smoothie: For a creamy, nutrient-dense smoothie, blend an avocado, banana, unsweetened chocolate powder, almond milk, and a spoonful of almond butter.

Recipes for Superfood Juice

1.Kale, spinach, cucumber, celery, green apple, and lemon can all be juiced to make a nutrient-rich green juice.

2.Carrot Ginger Juice: For an anti-inflammatory and immune-stimulating juice, juice carrots, ginger, apple, and lemon.

3.Beetroot Juice: For a heart-healthy and detoxifying juice, juice beets, carrots, apples, and ginger.

4.Citrus Boost Juice: For an anti-inflammatory and vitamin C-rich drink, juice oranges, grapefruits, lemons, and a small amount of turmeric.

Superfoods are a potent method to boost your nutrition and general well-being. You can give your body the vital nutrients it requires to function at its best and fend off disease by including a range of nutrient-dense foods in your daily routine, such as sea vegetables, berries, green leafy vegetables, turmeric, ginger, garlic, onions, and superfood smoothies and juices. In order to ensure that you receive a wide range of health advantages, it is important to adopt a diverse and balanced diet that contains a variety of these superfoods.

CHAPTER FOUR

ANTI-INFLAMMATORY DIET FOR CANCER PREVENTION

Cancer is one of the leading causes of death globally, and its prevention is a major focus in health and nutrition. One of the key strategies in cancer prevention is managing inflammation through diet. Chronic inflammation is linked to various types of cancer, and adopting an anti-inflammatory diet can help reduce this risk. This comprehensive guide explores the connection between inflammation and cancer, outlines the principles of an anti-inflammatory diet, provides a detailed list of foods to include and avoid, and offers sample meal plans and recipes to help maintain an anti-inflammatory lifestyle.

Understanding Inflammation and Cancer

What is Inflammation?

Inflammation is the body's natural response to injury or infection. It is a protective mechanism that involves the immune system releasing chemicals to fight off harmful stimuli and promote healing. There are two types of inflammation:

1. Acute Inflammation: This is a short-term response that occurs immediately after an injury or infection. Symptoms include redness, swelling, heat, and pain. Acute inflammation is essential for healing and typically resolves once the threat is eliminated.

2. Chronic Inflammation: This is a prolonged, low-grade inflammatory response that persists over time, often without an apparent injury or infection. Chronic inflammation can be detrimental to health, as it can damage tissues and organs, leading to various chronic diseases, including cancer.

The Link Between Inflammation and Cancer

Chronic inflammation is a major risk factor for cancer. It contributes to the development and progression of cancer in several ways:

1. DNA Damage: Inflammatory cells produce reactive oxygen species (ROS) and reactive nitrogen species (RNS), which can damage DNA, leading to mutations that increase the risk of cancer.

2. Cell Proliferation: Chronic inflammation promotes the proliferation of cells, including potentially cancerous cells, increasing the likelihood of tumor formation.

3. Angiogenesis: Inflammation stimulates the formation of new blood vessels (angiogenesis), which supply nutrients and oxygen to tumors, allowing them to grow and spread.

4. Immune Evasion: Chronic inflammation can suppress the immune system's ability to detect and destroy cancer cells, allowing tumors to evade immune surveillance.

Common Sources of Chronic Inflammation

Several factors can contribute to chronic inflammation, including:

1. Diet: A diet high in processed foods, sugars, and unhealthy fats can promote inflammation.

2. Lifestyle: Lack of exercise, smoking, and excessive alcohol consumption are major contributors.

3. Obesity: Excess body fat, especially around the abdomen, produces pro-inflammatory cytokines.

4. Chronic Infections: Persistent infections, such as hepatitis and human papillomavirus (HPV), can cause chronic inflammation.

5. Environmental Factors: Exposure to pollutants, toxins, and chemicals can trigger inflammatory responses.

KEY PRINCIPLES OF AN ANTI-INFLAMMATORY DIET

An anti-inflammatory diet focuses on reducing inflammation in the body through the consumption of nutrient-dense, whole foods. Here are the key principles:

1. Emphasize Whole Foods: Prioritize whole, unprocessed foods that are rich in nutrients and free from artificial additives.

2. Increase Antioxidants: Consume foods high in antioxidants, which neutralize free radicals and reduce oxidative stress.

3. Healthy Fats: Include sources of omega-3 fatty acids, which have anti-inflammatory properties, and limit omega-6 fatty acids and trans fats.

4. Fiber-Rich Foods: Incorporate plenty of fiber from fruits, vegetables, legumes, and whole grains to support gut health and reduce inflammation.

5. Limit Sugars and Refined Carbs: Reduce the intake of sugars and refined carbohydrates, which can spike blood sugar levels and promote inflammation.

6. Herbs and Spices: Use anti-inflammatory herbs and spices, such as turmeric, ginger, garlic, and cinnamon, to flavor foods.

7. Stay Hydrated: Drink plenty of water and avoid sugary drinks to maintain optimal hydration and support overall health.

FOODS TO INCLUDE FOR REDUCING INFLAMMATION

Incorporating a variety of anti-inflammatory foods into your diet can help reduce inflammation and lower the risk of cancer. Here are some key foods to include:

Fruits and Vegetables

1. Berries: Blueberries, strawberries, raspberries, and blackberries are rich in antioxidants, particularly anthocyanins, which reduce inflammation.

2. Leafy Greens: Spinach, kale, Swiss chard, and collard greens are high in vitamins, minerals, and antioxidants.

3. Cruciferous Vegetables: Broccoli, cauliflower, Brussels sprouts, and cabbage contain sulforaphane, which has anti-inflammatory properties.

4. Citrus Fruits: Oranges, lemons, and grapefruits are rich in vitamin C, which has antioxidant and anti-inflammatory effects.

5. Tomatoes: High in lycopene, an antioxidant that helps reduce inflammation.

Healthy Fats

1. Olive Oil: Rich in monounsaturated fats and polyphenols, olive oil has strong anti-inflammatory properties.

2. Avocados: High in healthy fats, fiber, and antioxidants.

3. Nuts and Seeds: Almonds, walnuts, flaxseeds, and chia seeds provide omega-3 fatty acids and other anti-inflammatory nutrients.

4. Fatty Fish: Salmon, mackerel, sardines, and anchovies are excellent sources of omega-3 fatty acids.

Whole Grains

1. Oats: Rich in fiber and antioxidants, oats help reduce inflammation.

2. Quinoa: A gluten-free grain high in protein, fiber, and antioxidants.

3. Brown Rice: A whole grain that provides fiber and essential nutrients.

Legumes

1. Lentils: High in fiber, protein, and antioxidants.

2. Chickpeas: Provide fiber, protein, and anti-inflammatory compounds.

3. Black Beans: Rich in fiber, protein, and phytonutrients.

Herbs and Spices

1. Turmeric: Contains curcumin, a powerful anti-inflammatory compound.

2. Ginger: Has anti-inflammatory and antioxidant properties.

3. Garlic: Contains sulfur compounds that reduce inflammation.

4. Cinnamon: Has anti-inflammatory and antioxidant effects.

Beverages

1. Green Tea: Rich in polyphenols, particularly epigallocatechin gallate (EGCG), which has anti-inflammatory properties.

2. Herbal Teas: Chamomile, ginger, and turmeric teas can help reduce inflammation.

FOODS TO AVOID FOR BETTER HEALTH

Certain foods can promote inflammation and should be limited or avoided in an anti-inflammatory diet:

Processed Foods

1. Processed Meats: Sausages, hot dogs, and deli meats contain preservatives and additives that promote inflammation.

2. Refined Grains: White bread, pasta, and pastries made from refined flour lack fiber and nutrients and can spike blood sugar levels.

3. Snack Foods: Chips, crackers, and other processed snacks often contain unhealthy fats and additives.

Sugars and Refined Carbohydrates

1. Sugary Beverages: Soda, energy drinks, and sweetened coffee drinks contain high amounts of sugar.

2. Sweets and Desserts: Candy, cookies, cakes, and pastries are high in sugar and refined carbs.

Unhealthy Fats

1. Trans Fats: Found in margarine, fried foods, and many processed snacks, trans fats are highly inflammatory.

2. Omega-6 Fatty Acids: While essential in small amounts, excessive intake from vegetable oils (corn, soybean, sunflower) can promote inflammation.

Red and Processed Meats

1. Red Meat: Beef, pork, and lamb can promote inflammation when consumed in excess.

2. Processed Meats: Bacon, sausages, and ham contain preservatives that can increase inflammation.

Artificial Additives

1. Artificial Sweeteners: Aspartame, sucralose, and other artificial sweeteners can disrupt gut health and promote inflammation.

2. Preservatives and Colorings: Additives in processed foods can trigger inflammatory responses.

Sample Meal Plans: Breakfast, Lunch, and Dinner

Breakfast

1. Berry Smoothie Bowl: Blend together a cup of mixed berries, a banana, a handful of spinach, and almond milk. Top with chia seeds, sliced almonds, and a drizzle of honey.

2. Overnight Oats: Combine rolled oats, almond milk, chia seeds, and a dash of cinnamon in a jar. Let it sit overnight in the refrigerator. In the morning, top with fresh berries and a dollop of Greek yogurt.

3. Avocado Toast: Spread mashed avocado on whole-grain toast. Top with cherry tomatoes, a sprinkle of chia seeds, and a drizzle of olive oil.

Lunch

1. Quinoa Salad: Mix cooked quinoa with chopped cucumbers, cherry tomatoes, red onion, and fresh parsley. Dress with lemon juice, olive oil, and a pinch of salt.

2. Lentil Soup: Cook lentils with diced carrots, celery, onions, and garlic in vegetable broth. Season with turmeric, cumin, and black pepper. Serve with a side of whole-grain bread.

3. Grilled Salmon and Veggies: Grill a salmon fillet seasoned with lemon and herbs. Serve with a side of steamed broccoli and roasted sweet potatoes.

Dinner

1. Stuffed Bell Peppers: Fill bell peppers with a mixture of cooked quinoa, black beans, corn, and diced tomatoes. Top with a sprinkle of cheese and bake until peppers are tender.

2. Chickpea and Spinach Curry: Sauté onions, garlic, and ginger in olive oil. Add chickpeas, spinach, diced tomatoes, and coconut milk. Season with curry powder, turmeric, and cumin. Serve with brown rice.

3. Veggie Stir-Fry: Stir-fry a mix of broccoli, bell peppers, carrots, and snap peas in olive oil. Add tofu or chicken and a sauce made from soy sauce, ginger, and garlic. Serve over quinoa or brown rice.

Anti-Inflammatory Recipes

Turmeric Ginger Smoothie

Ingredients:

- 1 banana
- 1 cup unsweetened almond milk
- 1/2 teaspoon ground turmeric
- 1/2 teaspoon ground ginger
- 1 tablespoon chia seeds
- 1 teaspoon honey or maple syrup (optional)

Instructions:

1. Combine all ingredients in a blender.
2. Blend until smooth.
3. Pour into a glass and enjoy.

Baked Salmon with Lemon and Dill

Ingredients:

- 4 salmon fillets
- 2 tablespoons olive oil
- 1 lemon, thinly sliced
- 1 tablespoon fresh dill, chopped

- Salt and pepper to taste

Instructions:

1. Preheat oven to 375°F (190°C).
2. Place salmon fillets on a baking sheet lined with parchment paper.
3. Drizzle olive oil over the fillets and season with salt and pepper.
4. Top with lemon slices and sprinkle with fresh dill.
5. Bake for 15-20 minutes, until salmon is cooked through.
6. Serve with a side of steamed vegetables.

Quinoa and Black Bean Salad

Ingredients:

- 1 cup quinoa, cooked and cooled
- 1 can black beans, rinsed and drained
- 1 red bell pepper, diced
- 1 avocado, diced
- 1/4 cup red onion, finely chopped
- 1/4 cup fresh cilantro, chopped
- Juice of 1 lime
- 2 tablespoons olive oil

- Salt and pepper to taste

Instructions:

1. In a large bowl, combine quinoa, black beans, bell pepper, avocado, red onion, and cilantro.
2. In a small bowl, whisk together lime juice, olive oil, salt, and pepper.
3. Pour dressing over the salad and toss to combine.
4. Serve immediately or refrigerate for later.

Turmeric and Ginger Chicken Soup

Ingredients:

- 1 tablespoon olive oil
- 1 onion, chopped
- 2 cloves garlic, minced
- 1 tablespoon fresh ginger, grated
- 1 teaspoon ground turmeric
- 4 cups chicken broth
- 2 cups cooked chicken, shredded
- 2 carrots, sliced
- 2 celery stalks, sliced
- 1 cup spinach

- Salt and pepper to taste

Instructions:

1. Heat olive oil in a large pot over medium heat.
2. Add onion, garlic, and ginger, and sauté until fragrant.
3. Add turmeric and stir to combine.
4. Pour in chicken broth and bring to a boil.
5. Add chicken, carrots, and celery, and reduce heat to simmer.
6. Cook for 15-20 minutes, until vegetables are tender.
7. Stir in spinach and season with salt and pepper.
8. Serve hot.

TIPS FOR MAINTAINING AN ANTI-INFLAMMATORY LIFESTYLE

1. Plan Your Meals: Prepare a weekly meal plan that includes a variety of anti-inflammatory foods. This will help you stay on track and avoid unhealthy choices.

2. Stay Hydrated: Drink plenty of water throughout the day to support overall health and reduce inflammation.

3. Exercise Regularly: Incorporate physical activity into your daily routine. Aim for at least 30 minutes of moderate exercise most days of the week.

4. Manage Stress: Practice stress-reducing techniques such as yoga, meditation, or deep breathing exercises to help lower inflammation.

5. Get Enough Sleep: Aim for 7-9 hours of quality sleep each night to support immune function and reduce inflammation.

6. Avoid Smoking and Excessive Alcohol: Both smoking and excessive alcohol consumption can promote inflammation and increase the risk of cancer.

7. Limit Exposure to Toxins: Reduce your exposure to environmental toxins by using natural cleaning products, avoiding plastics, and choosing organic foods when possible.

8. Regular Check-Ups: Schedule regular health check-ups and screenings to monitor your health and catch any potential issues early.

By understanding the connection between inflammation and cancer, and by adopting an anti-inflammatory diet and lifestyle, you can take proactive steps towards reducing your risk of cancer and promoting overall health. Incorporate a variety of nutrient-dense foods, avoid pro-inflammatory foods, and follow the tips for maintaining a healthy lifestyle to support your body's natural defenses and enhance your well-being.

CHAPTER FIVE

ALKALINE DIET: BALANCING YOUR BODY'S PH

The alkaline diet has been more well-known in recent years due to claims made by supporters that it can enhance wellbeing, encourage weight loss, and fend against chronic illnesses. In-depth discussions of the science underlying the alkaline diet, the idea of balancing the body's pH, the distinction between alkaline and acidic foods, potential health benefits, guidelines for preparing alkaline meals, sample daily meal plans, recipes for alkaline meals and snacks, and how to monitor and adjust your pH balance for optimal health are all included in this comprehensive guide.

The Alkaline Diet: The Science Behind It

The foundation of the alkaline diet is the idea that some foods have an impact on the pH levels of the body. The pH scale, which goes from 0 (extremely acidic) to 14 (very alkaline), with 7 being neutral, indicates how acidic or alkaline a substance is. The blood's pH in the human body is kept at a slightly alkaline 7.4, which is essential for healthy cells and general wellbeing.

Balance of Acid-Base

The body uses a number of methods, such as the following, to tightly manage its acid-base balance:

1. Buffers: By absorbing excess acids or bases, buffers are chemicals that aid in pH stabilization. Phosphate ions in the kidneys and bicarbonate ions in the blood are two examples.

2. Respiratory System: By modifying the blood's concentration of carbon dioxide (CO_2), the lungs control pH. Respiratory alkalosis is caused by low CO_2 levels, whereas respiratory acidosis is caused by high CO_2 levels.

3. Renal System: By eliminating bases and acids from the urine and reabsorbing bicarbonate ions, the kidneys are essential for preserving the acid-base balance.

THE THEORY OF ACID-ALKALINE

According to the acid-alkaline theory, the high acid content of modern diets, which include animal proteins, processed foods, and refined carbohydrates, can upset the pH balance of the body and cause chronic illnesses including cancer, kidney stones, and osteoporosis. Increased consumption of alkaline-forming foods, such as fruits, vegetables, and legumes, according to proponents of the alkaline diet, can aid in reestablishing equilibrium and enhancing health.

Criticism and Skepticism

The alkaline diet has grown in popularity, but it has also drawn criticism from nutrition experts and critics. Critics contend that dietary modifications have little effect on blood pH and that physiological processes closely control the body's pH. Additionally, they draw attention to the fact that an alkaline diet limits a number of nutritious items, including dairy, lean proteins, and whole grains, which, if improperly balanced, can result in vitamin deficiencies.

RECOGNIZING ACIDIC AND ALKALINE FOODS

Foods are categorized in the alkaline diet according to how much they can change the pH levels in the body. Foods are categorized as neutral, acidic, or alkaline-forming. Here's how these categories apply to several typical foods:

Foods That Form Alkaline

Foods that, after digestion, leave an alkaline residue in the body are said to be alkaline-forming. Usually, they contain minerals like calcium, magnesium, and potassium that act as pH balancers and acid buffers. As examples, consider:

- Fruits: Watermelon, bananas, avocados, berries (strawberries, blueberries, raspberries), and citrus fruits (lemons, limes, and oranges).

- Vegetables: Bell peppers, cauliflower, broccoli, cucumbers, celery, and leafy greens (kale, spinach, and Swiss chard).

- Legume: kidney, black, chickpeas, and lentils.

- Nuts and Seeds: Chia seeds, flaxseeds, walnuts, and almonds.

- Spices and Herbs: cinnamon, ginger, garlic, and turmeric.

Foods That Form An Acid

Foods that, when digested, leave an acidic residue in the body are considered acid-forming foods. They frequently contain phosphorus and amino acids that contain sulfur, which can enhance the generation of acid. Meat (beef, hog, lamb), poultry (chicken, turkey), fish, eggs, and dairy products (milk, cheese, yogurt) are a few examples of animal proteins.

• Processed Foods: packaged snacks (chips, cookies, crackers), refined grains (white bread, pasta, rice), sugar-filled drinks, and processed meats (bacon, sausage, deli meats).

• Fats and Oils: Fried foods, margarine, butter, and vegetable oils (soybean, corn, and sunflower).

Foods That Aren't Neutral

Foods classified as neutral have little effect on the pH of the body and are neither acidic nor alkaline-forming. As examples, consider:

• Whole Grains: millet, barley, quinoa, oats, and brown rice.

• Some proteins, such as beans, tempeh, and tofu (in moderation).

• Fats: Avocado, coconut, and olive oils.

• Drinks: Green tea, herbal teas, and water (in moderation).

Advantages of an Alkaline Diet for Health

The alkaline diet's proponents assert that it has several health advantages, such as:

1. Better Bone Health: Calcium and magnesium, which are vital for strong bones, are abundant in foods that generate an alkaline environment. The alkaline diet may help enhance bone density and prevent osteoporosis by lowering acid load.

2. Decreased Inflammation: Heart disease, diabetes, and cancer are just a few of the illnesses that are associated with chronic inflammation. Foods that create an alkaline environment have anti-inflammatory qualities and may aid in lowering bodily inflammation.

3. Weight Loss: The alkaline diet can help with weight loss and general health improvement by emphasizing full, nutrient-dense meals while reducing processed foods and sugars.

4. Better Digestion: Foods that generate an alkaline environment frequently contain a lot of fiber, which promotes digestive health and guards against constipation and other digestive problems.

5. Enhanced Energy: The alkaline diet may increase energy and lessen fatigue by encouraging a more alkaline environment in the body.

6. Enhanced Immunity: Foods that generate an alkaline environment are high in antioxidants, vitamins, and minerals that boost immunity and guard against illnesses and infections.

Further research is necessary to completely understand the impact of the alkaline diet on health and disease prevention, even if some studies have revealed possible benefits.

How to Make Alkaline Meals: A Guide and Some Advice

Developing alkaline meals entails reducing the amount of acidic-forming items in your diet and increasing the amount of alkaline-forming foods. Here are some rules and pointers for preparing meals that are alkaline:

1. Emphasis on Fruits and Vegetables: At each meal, place half of your plate on alkaline-forming fruits and vegetables. To make sure you receive a wide spectrum of nutrients, select a variety of colors and varieties.

2. Incorporate Leafy Greens: Because they are especially alkaline-forming, leafy greens like spinach, kale, and Swiss chard ought to be a regular component of your diet.

3. Select Plant-Based Proteins: Avoid animal proteins, which can cause acidity, and instead choose plant-based protein sources such legumes, tofu, and tempeh.

4. Use Healthy Fats: To counteract acidity, incorporate sources of healthy fats into your meals, such as avocados, nuts, seeds, and olive oil.

5. Reduce Processed Foods: Steer clear of extremely acidic and low-nutrient processed foods, refined grains, sugary snacks, and beverages.

6. Limit Animal Products: Since animal products can cause acidity, cut back on your consumption of meat, dairy, and eggs. If you do include them, go for organic, pasture-raised, and lean varieties.

7. Opt for Whole Grains: Unlike refined grains, whole grains like brown rice, quinoa, oats, and barley have lower acidity levels, so include them in your meals.

8. Drink A Lot of Water: Throughout the day, make sure you stay hydrated by consuming a lot of water. Water assists the body's

natural detoxification processes and aids in the removal of contaminants.

9. Balance Your Plate: Try to have a combination of foods that form an alkaline environment, good fats, and high-quality proteins on your plate. This will assist in giving your body the nourishment it requires to flourish. 10. Eat Slowly and Mindfully: To avoid overeating and aid in digestion, pay attention to your body's signals of hunger and fullness.

You may prepare balanced, alkaline meals that promote general health and well-being by adhering to these rules and recommendations.

Sample Daily Meal Plans

Here are two sample daily meal plans that incorporate alkaline-forming foods:

Sample Meal Plan 1:

Breakfast:

- Green Smoothie: Blend spinach, kale, banana, almond milk, and a scoop of plant-based protein powder.
- Whole Grain Toast: Top with mashed avocado, sliced tomatoes, and a sprinkle of hemp seeds.

Lunch:

- Quinoa Salad: Combine cooked quinoa with diced cucumbers, cherry tomatoes, bell peppers, black beans, and fresh cilantro. Dress with olive oil, lemon juice, and a pinch of salt.

- Mixed Berry Salad: Toss mixed berries (strawberries, blueberries, raspberries) with baby spinach, sliced almonds, and balsamic vinaigrette.

Dinner:

- Baked Salmon: Season salmon fillets with lemon juice, garlic, and dill. Bake until cooked through and serve with roasted asparagus and quinoa pilaf.
- Steamed Broccoli: Serve steamed broccoli drizzled with olive oil and seasoned with garlic powder and sea salt.

Snacks:

- Sliced Apple with Almond Butter
- Carrot Sticks with Hummus

Sample Meal Plan 2:

Breakfast:

- Overnight Oats: Combine rolled oats, chia seeds, almond milk, sliced bananas, and a dash of cinnamon in a jar. Let it sit overnight in the refrigerator. In the morning, top with fresh berries and a dollop of Greek yogurt.
- Green Tea

Lunch:

- Chickpea Salad: Mix chickpeas with diced cucumbers, cherry tomatoes, red onions, and fresh parsley. Dress with olive oil, lemon juice, and tahini. Serve over mixed greens.
- Quinoa Tabouli: Combine cooked quinoa with chopped parsley,tomatoes, cucumbers, and mint. Dress with lemon juice and olive oil.

Dinner:

- Stir-Fried Tofu and Vegetables: Stir-fry tofu with broccoli, bell peppers, snap peas, and mushrooms in a ginger-garlic sauce. Serve over brown rice.
- Steamed Green Beans: Steam green beans until tender-crisp and toss with lemon zest and toasted almonds.

Snacks:

- Greek Yogurt with Berries
- Trail Mix: Combine almonds, walnuts, pumpkin seeds, and dried cranberries.

Feel free to customize these meal plans based on your preferences and dietary needs. The key is to include a variety of alkaline-forming foods while minimizing acidic foods.

Recipes for Alkaline Meals and Snacks

Here are three recipes for alkaline meals and snacks that you can incorporate into your diet:

Recipe 1: Lemon-Garlic Roasted Vegetables

Ingredients:

- 1 head broccoli, cut into florets
- 2 bell peppers, sliced
- 1 red onion, sliced
- 3 cloves garlic, minced
- 2 tablespoons olive oil
- Juice of 1 lemon
- Salt and pepper to taste

Instructions:

1. Preheat the oven to 400°F (200°C).
2. In a large mixing bowl, combine the broccoli florets, bell peppers, red onion, minced garlic, olive oil, lemon juice, salt, and pepper. Toss until the vegetables are evenly coated.
3. Spread the vegetables in a single layer on a baking sheet lined with parchment paper.
4. Roast in the preheated oven for 20-25 minutes, or until the vegetables are tender and slightly caramelized.
5. Serve hot as a side dish or over quinoa for a complete meal.

Recipe 2: Mediterranean Chickpea Salad

Ingredients:

- 2 cups cooked chickpeas (or 1 can, drained and rinsed)
- 1 cucumber, diced

- 1 pint cherry tomatoes, halved
- 1/4 cup red onion, finely chopped
- 1/4 cup fresh parsley, chopped
- 2 tablespoons olive oil
- Juice of 1 lemon
- 1 teaspoon dried oregano
- Salt and pepper to taste

Instructions:

1. In a large mixing bowl, combine the chickpeas, diced cucumber, cherry tomatoes, red onion, and parsley.
2. In a small bowl, whisk together the olive oil, lemon juice, dried oregano, salt, and pepper to make the dressing.
3. Pour the dressing over the salad and toss until well combined.
4. Refrigerate for at least 30 minutes to allow the flavors to meld before serving.
5. Serve chilled as a refreshing salad or as a filling for pita pockets.

Recipe 3: Almond Butter Banana Smoothie

Ingredients:

- 1 ripe banana

- 1 cup unsweetened almond milk
- 2 tablespoons almond butter
- 1 tablespoon chia seeds
- 1 teaspoon honey or maple syrup (optional)
- 1/2 teaspoon vanilla extract
- Ice cubes (optional)

Instructions:

1. In a blender, combine the ripe banana, almond milk, almond butter, chia seeds, honey or maple syrup (if using), and vanilla extract.
2. If desired, add a handful of ice cubes to make the smoothie colder and thicker.
3. Blend until smooth and creamy, scraping down the sides of the blender as needed.
4. Pour the smoothie into glasses and serve immediately.

These recipes are not only delicious but also packed with alkaline-forming ingredients to support your body's pH balance and overall health.

Monitoring and Adjusting Your pH Balance

Although proponents of the alkaline diet assert that it can assist in preserving the body's natural pH balance, it is not always easy to measure and change pH levels. Blood pH is tightly regulated by the body through a number of buffering processes, thus dietary changes are unlikely to have a major impact.

Techniques for Measuring pH Balance

1. Urinary pH Testing: Those who advocate an alkaline diet suggest utilizing pH strips to measure the pH of urine. However, a number of variables, including nutrition, activity level, and hydration state, can cause variations in urine pH throughout the day. Urinary pH is not a good predictor of general health, even though it can offer some insight into acid-base balance.

2. Testing Blood pH: The body has a strict regulation over blood pH, which normally stays between 7.35 and 7.45. Usually, blood pH testing is limited to clinical settings where specific medical problems like acidosis or alkalosis need to be diagnosed.

Lifestyle Elements That Affect pH Harmony

Although eating has an effect on acid-base balance, various lifestyle choices can also affect the body's pH levels:

- Hydration: Keeping the right fluid and electrolyte balance, which aids in pH regulation, requires enough hydration.

- Stress: Prolonged stress can raise cortisol levels, which can have an impact on acid-base equilibrium.

- Physical Activity: Vigorous activity may cause the production of lactic acid, which momentarily lowers blood pH. On the other hand, consistent exercise is generally good for general health.

- Sleep: Inadequate or poor quality sleep can upset metabolic and hormonal balance, which may have an impact on pH regulation.

• Medication Use: Some drugs, such steroids and diuretics, might alter acid-base balance and may need to be closely watched by a medical expert.

Advice for Maintaining pH Balance

Although it might not be feasible or required to maintain a particular pH level, there are actions you can do to promote general health and wellbeing:

1. Eat a Balanced Diet: To promote general health, concentrate on consuming a range of whole, nutrient-dense foods, including an abundance of fruits and vegetables.

2. Stay Hydrated: To support optimal fluid balance and hydration, consume a sufficient amount of water throughout the day.

3. Control Stress: To encourage relaxation and general well-being, engage in stress-reduction practices like yoga, deep breathing exercises, or meditation.

4. Get Regular Exercise: Exercise on a regular basis to preserve muscle mass, improve cardiovascular health, and enhance general vigor.

5. Make Sleep a Priority: To maintain immunological response, hormonal balance, and metabolic health, aim for 7-9 hours of good sleep per night.

6. Reduce Toxin Exposure: Eat organic foods, use natural household and personal care products, and cut less on plastics to reduce your exposure to environmental toxins and pollutants.

7. Seek Professional counsel: For individualized counsel and guidance, speak with a healthcare provider if you have concerns about your pH balance or general health.

Through an emphasis on holistic lifestyle components and the integration of healthful practices into your everyday regimen, you can bolster your body's innate capacity to preserve ideal pH equilibrium and advance general health and wellness.

In summary, there is scant scientific evidence to support the effectiveness of the alkaline diet, despite the fact that it stresses the consumption of alkaline-forming foods to support the body's pH equilibrium. On the other hand, increasing your intake of fruits, vegetables, and plant-based foods can have a number of positive effects on your health, such as better digestion, more energy, and a decrease in inflammation. To support general health and well-being, it is important to focus on whole, minimally processed foods and adopt good lifestyle practices. You can choose to follow the alkaline diet or just prioritize a balanced, nutrient-rich diet.

CHAPTER SIX

KETO-DIETARY APPROACHES TO CANCER TREATMENT

The ketogenic diet has drawn interest as a possible treatment strategy for treating cancer in addition to being a tool for weight loss. This thorough book examines the ketogenic diet in relation to managing cancer. It covers the diet's principles, mechanisms of action, suggested foods, techniques for meal planning, examples of meal plans and recipes, handling of side effects, and long-term issues.

The Ketogenic Diet: What Is It?

A high-fat, low-carb diet called the ketogenic diet has been used for decades to treat childhood epilepsy. It entails cutting back on carbohydrates considerably and substituting moderate amounts of protein and healthy fats. The main objective of the ketogenic diet is to bring the body into a metabolic state called ketosis, where it starts using ketones—which are made from fat in the liver—instead of glucose as its main energy source.

Fundamentals of a Ketogenic Diet:

1. Low Carbohydrate Intake: The daily allowance of carbohydrates is limited to fewer than 50 grams, or 5–10% of total calories.

2. Moderate Protein Intake: To avoid excessive gluconeogenesis, or the conversion of protein into glucose, the daily caloric intake of protein should be moderate, including approximately 15-20% of total calories.

3. High Fat Intake: Healthy fats, which account for 70–75% of daily calories, provide the majority of calories.

4. Inducing Ketosis: The body enters a state of ketosis when fat intake is increased and carbs are restricted. In this state, ketone bodies take over as the main energy source for all cells, including cancer cells.

How Cancer Is Fought by Ketosis

The capacity of the ketogenic diet to target metabolic pathways that are dysregulated in cancer cells has drawn attention to it as a possible supplementary therapy for managing cancer. The following pathways could account for ketosis's anti-cancer effects:

1. Starving Cancer Cells: To support their explosive growth and multiplication, cancer cells have a high glucose requirement. The ketogenic diet may starve cancer cells and prevent them from growing and spreading by lowering glucose availability and carbohydrate intake.

2. Modifying Cellular Metabolism: The body creates ketone bodies during ketosis as a substitute for glucose as a fuel source. Many cancer cells, in contrast to normal cells, have abnormalities in their mitochondria and, even in the presence of oxygen, predominantly rely on glycolysis—the process of converting glucose into energy—for energy generation (a phenomenon known as the Warburg

effect). Cancer cells may use ketones less effectively, which could put them at a metabolic disadvantage and possibly stop their proliferation.

3. Reducing Inflammation: The onset and spread of cancer are both influenced by chronic inflammation. In preclinical and clinical research, the ketogenic diet has been demonstrated to lower inflammatory markers, which may help make the environment less conducive to the formation of cancer.

4. Increasing Autophagy: Autophagy is a biological process that aids in the removal of damaged proteins and organelles, fostering cellular survival and renewal. According to some research, the ketogenic diet may improve autophagy, which may have anticancer effects by removing cellular debris and encouraging the death of cancerous cells.

5. Increasing Sensitivity to Insulin: A hormone called insulin controls blood sugar levels and encourages cell division. Insulin resistance has been connected to a higher risk of developing several malignancies and is frequently linked to obesity and high-carb diets. The ketogenic diet may decrease insulin levels and increase insulin sensitivity, which may lessen the risk and progression of cancer.

Brain tumors, breast cancer, and pancreatic cancer are just a few of the cancer types for which preclinical research and early clinical trials have produced encouraging results, however the evidence for using the ketogenic diet to treat cancer is still developing. To clarify the best dietary practices, possible adverse effects, and long-term consequences of ketogenic therapy in cancer patients, more research is necessary.

Low-Carb, High-Fat Foods to Incorporate

On the ketogenic diet, it's critical to eat foods high in good fats and low in carbohydrates in order to enter ketosis. Here are a few food examples to consider:

Good Fats:

1. Avocado: An essential component of the ketogenic diet, avocados are high in fiber and monounsaturated fats.

2. Coconut Oil: Rich in medium-chain triglycerides (MCTs), the liver easily transforms coconut oil into ketones.

3. Olive Oil: Rich in antioxidants and monounsaturated fats, olive oil is great for low-temperature cooking and salad dressings.

4. Nuts and Seeds: Packed with fiber, necessary nutrients, and good fats, almonds, walnuts, macadamia nuts, chia seeds, and flaxseeds are a great source of nutrition.

5. Fatty Fish: Omega-3 fatty acids, which have anti-inflammatory qualities, are abundant in salmon, mackerel, sardines, and trout.

6. Grass-fed butter and ghee: These are better sources of saturated fats than processed spreads and margarine.

7. Full-Fat Dairy: In moderation, high-fat dairy products like cheese, cream, and full-fat yogurt can be consumed.

8. Eggs: Packed with protein and good fats, eggs are a nutrient-dense and adaptable food.

Low-Carb Produce:

1. Leafy Greens: Rich in fiber, vitamins, and minerals, leafy greens such as spinach, kale, and Swiss chard are low in carbs.

2. Cruciferous Vegetables: Brussels sprouts, cabbage, cauliflower, and broccoli are low in carbohydrates and high in nutrients.

3. Summer squash: Low in carbohydrates, zucchini and other squashes can be spiralized to make keto-friendly noodles.

4. Bell peppers: These colorful and flavorful additions to food have a low carbohydrate content.

5. Asparagus: Low in carbohydrates, asparagus goes well with foods high in protein.

6. Mushrooms: You may use mushrooms in a variety of keto-friendly recipes because they are low in carbohydrates.

7. Cucumber: Cucumbers are a low-carb, hydrating veggie that tastes good both pickled and raw.

You can design a ketogenic diet plan that supports ketosis and might be beneficial for managing cancer by concentrating on these high-fat, low-carb meals.

Meal Planning for Keto Dieters

Meal planning for keto requires choosing foods that are low in carbohydrates, moderate in protein, and rich in healthy fats. The following advice can help you organize ketogenic meals:

1. Put an emphasis on Whole Foods: Opt for nutrient-dense, whole foods like avocados, fatty fish, nuts, seeds, and non-starchy veggies.

2. Include a Protein Source: Add a protein-rich food to every meal, such as cheese, eggs, fish, poultry, or tofu.

3. Add Good Fats: To reach your recommended daily intake of fat, include foods and drinks that are high in healthy fats, such as butter, avocado, coconut, and olive oil.

4. Reduce Carbohydrates: Cut back on foods heavy in carbohydrates, such as grains, fruits, vegetables with a lot of starch, and sugary snacks and drinks.

5. Experiment with Recipes: Use your imagination in the kitchen to find ideas for keto-friendly dishes. Ideas for ketogenic meals can be found in a plethora of web resources.

6. Meal Prep: To save time and make sure you have keto-friendly options on hand all week, think about meal planning. For quick and easy meals, prepare keto-friendly snacks and meals ahead of time, portion them into containers, and keep them in the freezer or refrigerator.

7. Examine Labels: Pay attention to food labels and select those devoid of refined grains, added sugars, and low in carbs. Whenever possible, choose whole, minimally processed foods.

8. Remain Hydrated: To help with metabolic processes and to stay hydrated, sip lots of water throughout the day. Additionally, some people might benefit from including electrolyte-rich drinks like bone broth or electrolyte supplements, particularly in the beginning stages of switching to a ketogenic diet.

Pay Attention to Your Body: Observe your body's reaction to the ketogenic diet. While some people may feel invigorated and intellectually bright at first, others may experience immediate adverse effects like headaches, lethargy, or intestinal problems. Adapt your food consumption to your unique requirements and nutritional preferences.

10. Speak with a Medical Expert: It is imperative that you speak with a healthcare provider before beginning any new diet, especially one as restrictive as the ketogenic diet, especially if you are taking medication or have underlying medical conditions. To make sure the diet is secure and suitable for you, they can offer you individualized advice and track your development.

Sample Ketogenic Meal Plans and Recipes

Here are two sample ketogenic meal plans, along with accompanying recipes, to provide you with inspiration for incorporating keto-friendly meals into your diet:

Sample Meal Plan 1:

Breakfast:

- Keto Avocado and Egg Breakfast Bowl

    - Ingredients: Avocado, eggs, spinach, cherry tomatoes, olive oil, salt, pepper.
    - Instructions: Slice an avocado in half and remove the pit. Scoop out some of the flesh to create a larger cavity. Crack an egg into each avocado half. Place the avocados on a

baking sheet, add spinach and halved cherry tomatoes to the tray, drizzle everything with olive oil, and season with salt and pepper. Bake in a preheated oven at 375°F (190°C) for 15-20 minutes or until the eggs are cooked to your liking.

Lunch:

- Keto Chicken Caesar Salad

    - Ingredients: Grilled chicken breast, romaine lettuce, Parmesan cheese, Caesar dressing (made with olive oil, anchovies, garlic, Dijon mustard, lemon juice, and Parmesan cheese).

    - Instructions: Chop romaine lettuce and place it in a bowl. Add sliced grilled chicken breast, shaved Parmesan cheese, and homemade Caesar dressing. Toss everything together until well coated.

Dinner:

- Keto Salmon with Asparagus

    - Ingredients: Salmon fillet, asparagus spears, lemon, olive oil, salt, pepper, garlic powder.

    - Instructions: Place salmon fillets and asparagus spears on a baking sheet. Drizzle with olive oil, squeeze fresh lemon juice over the top, and season with salt, pepper, and garlic powder. Bake in a preheated oven at 400°F (200°C) for 12-15 minutes or until the salmon is cooked through and the asparagus is tender.

Snacks:

- Keto Cheese and Pepperoni
- Keto Avocado Deviled Eggs

Sample Meal Plan 2:

Breakfast:

- Keto Coconut Chia Pudding
    - Ingredients: Chia seeds, unsweetened coconut milk, vanilla extract, unsweetened shredded coconut, stevia or erythritol (optional).
    - Instructions: Mix chia seeds, coconut milk, and vanilla extract in a bowl. Sweeten to taste with stevia or erythritol, if desired. Let the mixture sit in the refrigerator for at least 2 hours or overnight until it thickens into a pudding-like consistency. Serve topped with shredded coconut.

Lunch:

- Keto Cobb Salad
    - Ingredients: Mixed greens, grilled chicken breast, bacon, hard-boiled eggs, avocado, blue cheese, cherry tomatoes, ranch dressing (made with mayonnaise, sour cream, garlic powder, onion powder, dried parsley, dried dill, and apple cider vinegar).
    - Instructions: Arrange mixed greens in a bowl. Top with sliced grilled chicken breast, crumbled bacon, sliced hard-boiled eggs, diced avocado, crumbled blue cheese, and halved cherry tomatoes. Drizzle with homemade ranch dressing.

Dinner:

- Keto Beef and Broccoli Stir-Fry

    - Ingredients: Beef sirloin, broccoli florets, garlic, ginger, soy sauce or coconut aminos, sesame oil, erythritol or stevia (optional), green onions, sesame seeds.

    - Instructions: Slice beef sirloin thinly and marinate in a mixture of minced garlic, grated ginger, soy sauce or coconut aminos, sesame oil, and a sweetener such as erythritol or stevia (optional). Stir-fry the beef in a hot skillet until browned, then add broccoli florets and continue cooking until tender. Serve garnished with sliced green onions and sesame seeds.

Snacks:

- Keto Almond Butter Fat Bombs
- Keto Veggie Sticks with Guacamole

These sample meal plans and recipes demonstrate how diverse and flavorful ketogenic meals can be while adhering to the principles of the ketogenic diet.

Managing Side Effects of the Ketogenic Diet

The ketogenic diet might have adverse effects, just like any other dietary intervention, especially in the early stages of the shift. The following list of typical ketogenic diet side effects includes management techniques for each:

1.Keto Flu: In the initial days or weeks after beginning a ketogenic diet, some people may experience flu-like symptoms such as headaches, nausea, irritability, lethargy, and dizziness. This occurrence, also referred to as the "keto flu," is usually temporary and can be avoided by drinking plenty of water, rehydrating, and gradually introducing electrolytes (sodium, potassium, and magnesium) into your diet instead of dramatically cutting off carbohydrates.

2.Digestive Problems: Constipation, diarrhea, or bloating are examples of digestive problems that can occasionally result from changes in the amount of dietary fiber consumed and the makeup of the gut microbiota. These symptoms can be lessened by increasing the amount of fiber you get from low-carb veggies, including fermented foods like kimchi or sauerkraut, and drinking plenty of water.

3.Electrolyte Imbalance: Because the ketogenic diet increases the excretion of sodium, potassium, and magnesium, it can cause electrolyte abnormalities. Think about taking electrolyte supplements, eating foods high in electrolytes, such avocados and leafy greens, and adding salt to food to prevent deficits.

4.Electrolyte abnormalities, dehydration, and modifications in muscular glycogen reserves can all lead to cramping in the muscles. Muscle cramps can be avoided or lessened with proper hydration, electrolyte consumption, and a gradual transition to a ketogenic food regime.

5.Fatigue: As the body adjusts to using ketones as its main fuel source, some people may feel fatigued, particularly in the early stages of a ketogenic diet. Fatigue can be lessened by getting enough sleep, staying hydrated, eating a balanced diet, and using electrolytes.

6.Changes in Exercise Performance: When switching to a ketogenic diet, athletes and active people may notice changes in their ability to perform, especially during high-intensity or anaerobic exercises that depend on glycogen storage. Although some individuals adjust to keto-adapted exercise effectively, others might gain from consuming certain amounts of carbohydrates prior to, during, or following workouts.

7.Levels of Lipid and Cholesterol: The ketogenic diet may cause alterations in lipid and cholesterol, such as a rise in low-density lipoprotein (LDL) and a fall in triglycerides. Even though these changes are usually temporary and don't always signify negative health consequences, it's crucial to routinely check lipid profiles, particularly in people who already have cardiovascular risk factors.

8.Social Difficulties: Eating a ketogenic diet can be socially awkward, particularly when dining out or in social situations when foods high in carbohydrates are popular. You can handle social situations more easily if you prepare ahead of time, let friends and family know what you eat, and concentrate on keto-friendly foods.

9.Emotional and Psychological Impact: Strict eating regimens, like the ketogenic diet, can occasionally cause emotions of loneliness, annoyance, or worry, particularly if sticking to them becomes difficult or if social contacts are hampered. During your ketogenic journey, seeking out emotional and psychological assistance from healthcare professionals, online networks, or support groups might be beneficial.

10. Medical Considerations: People who suffer from pancreatitis, gallbladder illness, liver disease, or metabolic abnormalities should be very cautious when implementing the ketogenic diet, or they should avoid it completely. Before beginning any new diet, it is imperative to speak with a healthcare provider, particularly if you are using medication or have underlying health issues.

The benefits of the ketogenic diet can be maximized while any negative effects are minimized by being aware of these possible side effects and putting methods in place to handle them.

Long-Term Advantages and Things to Think About

Although there is potential for the ketogenic diet to be a therapeutic method in the management of cancer and other health disorders, it is important to take into account potential long-term benefits and drawbacks.

1. Weight management: Studies have linked the ketogenic diet to benefits in body composition, such as decreased body fat and preserved lean muscle mass, as well as weight loss. Long-term weight management objectives may be supported by the ketogenic diet since it increases satiety and stabilizes blood sugar levels.

2. Metabolic Health: Studies have demonstrated improvements in lipid profiles, insulin sensitivity, and blood sugar regulation as indicators of metabolic health when following a ketogenic diet. Long-term benefits for lowering the risk of obesity, type 2 diabetes, and cardiovascular disease may result from these metabolic improvements.

3.Brain Health: New research indicates that the ketogenic diet may offer advantages for brain health, including neuroprotective effects. The production of ketones during ketosis may offer the brain an alternate fuel source, which may be helpful for diseases including epilepsy, Parkinson's, Alzheimer's, and traumatic brain damage.

4.Cancer treatment: Targeting metabolic pathways that are dysregulated in cancer cells, preliminary evidence suggests that the ketogenic diet may offer potential benefits for cancer treatment, while additional research is necessary. Based on specific findings, the ketogenic diet may prolong lifespan in some cancer populations, improve quality of life, and increase the effectiveness of traditional cancer treatments.

5.Lifestyle Sustainability: Because the ketogenic diet is so rigorous and may have social repercussions, some people may find it difficult to follow it for an extended period of time. However, many people find the ketogenic diet to be a pleasant and sustainable lifestyle choice when they combine flexibility, careful meal planning, and support from peers and healthcare experts.

6.Individual Variation: It's important to understand that different people will react differently to the ketogenic diet. Individual characteristics can impact the efficacy and acceptability of the ketogenic diet for long-term use, including genetics, metabolic health, exercise level, and personal preferences. Discovering the eating strategy that is most effective for you requires self-awareness and experimentation.

7.Nutritional Adequacy: Because of the diet's restriction, there may be a chance of nutrient deficiencies when following a ketogenic diet. Focus on eating a range of nutrient-dense meals, such as high-quality protein sources, low-carb veggies, and healthy fats, to maintain nutritional sufficiency. To satisfy your micronutrient requirements, think about consuming meals or supplements that have been fortified.

8.Frequent Monitoring: If you decide to stick to a ketogenic diet over the long term, it's critical to keep an eye on your health and seek medical advice as necessary. Frequent examinations, blood tests, and nutritional status evaluations can assist make sure you're reaching your health objectives and spot any possible problems early on.

In conclusion, by focusing on metabolic pathways that are dysregulated in disease states, the ketogenic diet holds potential as a therapeutic strategy for treating cancer and other medical disorders. You can maximize the potential advantages of the ketogenic diet for your health and well-being by concentrating on high-fat, low-carb foods, organizing balanced meals, controlling side effects, and taking long-term benefits and considerations into account. Like any diet, the ketogenic diet should be followed carefully. You should also tailor your plan to your own requirements and preferences and consult a healthcare provider as needed.

CHAPTER SEVEN

CONSUMING A PLANT-BASED DIET: FUELING YOUR BODY

The plant-based diet has become more and more well-liked in recent years due to its many health advantages and favorable effects on the environment. The advantages of a plant-based diet, vital nutrients found in plant-based foods, sources of protein for vegetarians and vegans, methods for preparing balanced plant-based meals, mouthwatering recipes to try, typical problems faced by plant-based eaters, and motivational success stories of people who have made the switch are all covered in this extensive guide.

advantages of a diet high in plants

Whole, minimally processed plant foods—such as fruits, vegetables, grains, legumes, nuts, and seeds—are the focus of a plant-based diet. The following are some of the main advantages of a plant-based diet:

1.Better Heart Health: Diets strong in fiber, antioxidants, and phytonutrients, and naturally low in cholesterol and saturated fat, can help lower blood pressure, lessen inflammation, and reduce the risk of heart disease.

2.Reduced Risk of Chronic Diseases: Studies indicate that eating a plant-based diet may lower your chance of developing long-term conditions like type 2 diabetes, high blood pressure, several malignancies, and obesity. Plant meals are rich in vitamins, minerals, and antioxidants that promote general health and may help avert the onset of chronic illnesses.

3.Weight management: Diets based primarily on plants tend to be higher in fiber and lower in calories than diets high in animal products. They may therefore enhance satiety, encourage weight loss, and assist long-term weight management objectives.

4.Digestive Health: Plant-based meals' high fiber content helps to maintain regularity in the digestive system, avoid constipation, and support healthy gut flora. A diet high in whole grains, legumes, fruits, and vegetables helps support the upkeep of a healthy digestive tract.

5.Environmental Sustainability: Diets high in plant-based foods are less harmful to the environment than those high in animal products. Producing plant foods uses less natural resources, such as land and water, produces less greenhouse gas emissions, and lessens habitat degradation and deforestation.

6.Animal Welfare: Eating a plant-based diet lowers the need for animal products and promotes moral and environmentally friendly agricultural methods. Plant-based diets lessen animal suffering and advance animal welfare, which are values that are consistent with compassion and respect for animals.

7.Longevity: Research has indicated that a plant-based diet may be linked to a longer lifetime and a decreased chance of passing away too soon from all causes. Plant-based diets increase longevity and vitality by lowering the risk of chronic diseases and increasing general health.

Vital Elements in Plant-Based Diets

If a plant-based diet is combined with variety and balance, it can supply your body with all the critical elements it needs for maximum health. The following are important nutrients that can be obtained through diet from plant-based foods:

1. Legumes (beans, lentils, chickpeas), tofu, tempeh, edamame, seitan, nuts, seeds, and whole grains (quinoa, barley, brown rice) are plant-based sources of protein. You can be sure you're getting all the important amino acids your body requires by combining different plant-based protein sources throughout the day.

2. Calcium: For plant-based diets, fortified plant milks (such almond, soy, or oat milk), tofu that has been fortified with calcium sulfate, leafy greens (like bok choy, collard greens, or kale), almonds, and sesame seeds are good sources of calcium.

3. Iron: Legumes, chickpeas, tofu, tempeh, fortified cereals, quinoa, pumpkin seeds, spinach, and dried apricots are plant-based sources of iron. Vitamin C-rich foods like tomatoes, bell peppers, and citrus fruits can improve the absorption of iron from plant-based diets.

4. Omega-3 Fatty Acids: Flaxseeds, chia seeds, hemp seeds, walnuts, and algae-based supplements are plant-based sources of omega-3 fatty acids. Consuming these items on a daily basis can help you guarantee that you are getting enough omega-3 fatty acids, which are critical for heart and brain function.

5. Vitamin B12: Since animal products are the main source of vitamin B12, it's critical for vegans and vegetarians to get their B12

from fortified foods including plant milks, cereals for breakfast, nutritional yeast, and supplements.

6.Vitamin D: In addition to being produced by the body when exposed to sunshine, vitamin D can also be acquired from supplements and fortified foods including cereals, orange juice, and plant milks. For plant-based diets, UV-exposed mushrooms provide a natural source of vitamin D.

7.Zinc: Legumes, nuts, seeds, whole grains, tofu, tempeh, and fortified breakfast cereals are plant-based sources of zinc. The absorption of zinc can be improved by soaking, sprouting, or fermenting grains and legumes.

8.Seaweed and iodized salt are the main sources of iodine. You can meet your iodine needs on a plant-based diet by using iodized salt or by include iodine-rich seaweed, such as kombu, wakame, or nori, in your diet.

You can make sure you're meeting your nutritional needs and promoting general health and well-being by including a range of nutrient-rich plant foods in your diet.

Vegetarian Sources of Protein

Protein is a necessary macronutrient that is vital for immune system support, tissue growth and repair, and the maintenance of muscular mass and strength. Even while meat is frequently thought of as the main source of protein in the diet, there are many plant-based protein sources that can give your body all the critical amino acids it requires. Here are some vegan and vegetarian dishes that are high in protein:

1.Legumes: A great source of plant-based protein are legumes, which include beans, lentils, chickpeas, and peas. They are a wholesome complement to any plant-based diet because they are also high in fiber, vitamins, and minerals. A range of legumes can be used in your meals; try using chickpeas in salads, black beans in tacos, and lentils in soups.

2.Tofu: A versatile plant-based source of protein, tofu, sometimes called bean curd, is manufactured from soybeans. Its mild flavor makes it versatile in many cooking applications, such as smoothies, scrambles, curries, and stir-fries. There are several textures of tofu, including silken, soft, firm, and extra firm, so you can select the one that works best for your recipe.

3.Tempeh: Tempeh is a rich, chewy, nutty-flavored food made from fermented soybeans. With regard to completeness, it includes all nine necessary amino acids. Tempeh can be used as a meat alternative in sandwiches, tacos, and stir-fries by marinating, grilling, crumbling, or stir-frying it.

4.Edamame: Young soybeans that are picked before reaching full maturity are known as edamame. Usually served hot or cold in their pods, with a dash of salt, as a snack or appetizer. To increase the protein value of salads, stir-fries, and pasta meals, edamame can be added.

5.Seitan: Made from gluten, the primary protein found in wheat, seitan is often referred to as wheat gluten or wheat meat. It can be seasoned and cooked in a variety of ways, including frying, baking, or boiling in broth. Its texture is chewy. Due to its high protein content and meat-like texture, seitan is especially well-liked in vegetarian and vegan dishes.

6.Legumes: Legumes are available in a variety of hues, including as green, brown, red, and black. They bring nutrition and taste to soups, stews, salads, and grain bowls since they are high in protein, fiber, and iron. While green and brown lentils retain their shape well when cooked, red lentils cook more quickly and have a softer texture.

7.Garbanzo beans, sometimes referred to as chickpeas, are a versatile legume that are frequently used in Middle Eastern and Mediterranean cooking. They can be boiled and added to salads, soups, curries, and wraps for an extra protein boost. They can also be roasted and seasoned for a crunchy snack or mashed into hummus.

8.Quinoa: Rich in protein, fiber, and vital elements, quinoa is a naturally gluten-free pseudo-cereal. It is a comprehensive source of protein since it includes all nine essential amino acids. When cooked, quinoa can be added to salads, eaten as a side dish, or used as the foundation for dishes like stuffed peppers, grain bowls, and porridge for breakfast.

9.Nuts and Seeds: Packed full of protein, good fats, vitamins, and minerals, nuts and seeds are foods high in nutrients. Plant-based protein sources include almonds, peanuts, cashews, walnuts, chia seeds, flaxseeds, hemp seeds, pumpkin seeds, and sunflower seeds. They can be added to salads, cereal, yogurt, or enjoyed as a snack when raw or roasted. They can also be used to produce nut butters, seed crackers, and energy bars.

10.Soy Products: There are a number of soy-based products available besides tempeh and tofu, including soy yogurt, soy cheese, soy milk, and soy meat alternatives including veggie burgers, sausages, and deli slices. These items offer a simple supply of plant-based protein and can be substituted for dairy and meat in recipes.

You can make sure you're fulfilling your protein requirements while eating tasty and nourishing meals by incorporating a range of these plant-based protein sources into your diet.

Making Plant-Based Meals That Are Balanced

A range of nutrient-rich foods from all dietary groups, such as fruits, vegetables, whole grains, legumes, nuts, and seeds, must be included when preparing balanced plant-based meals. The following advice can help you create well-balanced plant-based meals:

1.Begin with a Base: For your meal, select a nutrient-dense base such leafy greens (spinach, kale, arugula), whole grains (brown rice, quinoa, barley), or starchy vegetables (sweet potatoes, squash, corn).

2.Add Protein: You can add beans, lentils, tofu, tempeh, edamame, chickpeas, or quinoa to your meal as a plant-based source of protein. For the purpose of maintaining muscular health, fullness, and general nutrition, try to include protein with every meal.

3.Include Vegetables: To give your dish color, flavor, and texture, load it up with non-starchy vegetables. Add a range of veggies, including leafy greens, bell peppers, carrots, cucumbers, tomatoes, and mushrooms. Cruciferous vegetables include broccoli, cauliflower, and Brussels sprouts.

4.Include Healthy Fats: To promote nutrient absorption, cognitive function, and satiety, include sources of healthy fats in your meals. Add avocado slices, dress your salad or veggies with olive oil or tahini, garnish your food with nuts or seeds, or use olives or coconut milk in your recipes.

5.Enhance Flavor and Seasoning: Use herbs, spices, and condiments to bring out the flavors in your plant-based meals. To make tasty and filling meals, try experimenting with different seasonings like garlic, ginger, turmeric, cumin, paprika, basil, cilantro, and lemon juice.

6.Incorporate entire meals: Whenever feasible, give priority to entire, minimally processed meals. Make your own sauces, dressings, and marinades to keep ingredients under control and steer clear of extra sugars and bad fats. Go for fresh or frozen fruits and vegetables over canned or processed ones.

7.Balanced Macronutrients: To promote general health and long-lasting energy, try to incorporate the right amounts of fat, protein, and carbohydrates in each meal. Macronutrient balancing can aid in promoting satiety, preventing energy crashes, and stabilizing blood sugar levels.

8.Practice Portion Control: Keep an eye on serving sizes to prevent overindulging and make sure you're getting all the nutrients you need without going overboard on calories. For each food group, estimate the proper portion sizes using measuring cups, spoons, or visual cues.

9.Keep Yourself Hydrated: To stay hydrated and promote healthy digestion, metabolism, and general health, sip lots of water throughout the day. In addition to being hydrating, herbal teas, infused water, and coconut water can help vary your beverage selections.

10. Listen to Your Body: Be aware of your body's signals of hunger and fullness as well as the effects that various foods have on your mood. Chew carefully, eat with awareness, and enjoy the tastes and sensations of your food. Pay attention to your body's signals of hunger and fullness when choosing foods and adjusting portion sizes.

You may make tasty, filling, and nutritious plant-based meals that promote your general health and well-being by according to these suggestions.

Delicious Plant-Based Recipes

Here are some delicious and nutritious plant-based recipes to inspire you in the kitchen:

Breakfast:

1. Avocado Toast with Chickpea Salad:
    - Ingredients: Whole grain bread, ripe avocado, canned chickpeas, cherry tomatoes, cucumber, red onion, lemon juice, olive oil, salt, pepper.
    - Instructions: Mash avocado onto toasted whole grain bread. In a bowl, mix drained and rinsed chickpeas with diced tomatoes, cucumber, and red onion. Dress with lemon juice, olive oil, salt, and pepper. Spoon the chickpea salad over the avocado toast and enjoy!

2. Berry Smoothie Bowl:

    - Ingredients: Frozen mixed berries, banana, spinach or kale, almond milk, chia seeds, granola, fresh fruit (such as sliced banana, strawberries, or blueberries), almond butter or peanut butter (optional).

    - Instructions: Blend frozen berries, banana, spinach or kale, and almond milk until smooth. Pour into a bowl and top with chia seeds, granola, fresh fruit, and a drizzle of almond butter or peanut butter, if desired.

Lunch:

1. Mediterranean Quinoa Salad:

    - Ingredients: Cooked quinoa, cherry tomatoes, cucumber, red onion, Kalamata olives, fresh parsley, lemon juice, olive oil, salt, pepper.

    - Instructions: In a large bowl, combine cooked quinoa with halved cherry tomatoes, diced cucumber, sliced red onion, chopped Kalamata olives, and chopped fresh parsley. Dress with lemon juice, olive oil, salt, and pepper. Toss everything together until well combined and serve chilled.

2. Vegan Buddha Bowl:

    - Ingredients: Cooked brown rice or quinoa, roasted sweet potatoes, steamed broccoli, sautéed kale or spinach, avocado slices, chickpeas (roasted or sautéed), tahini dressing (tahini, lemon juice, garlic, water, salt).

- Instructions: Arrange cooked rice or quinoa, roasted sweet potatoes, steamed broccoli, sautéed kale or spinach, avocado slices, and chickpeas in a bowl. Drizzle with tahini dressing and garnish with sesame seeds or fresh herbs.

Dinner:

1. Vegetable Stir-Fry with Tofu:

    - Ingredients: Extra-firm tofu, mixed vegetables (such as bell peppers, broccoli, carrots, snap peas), garlic, ginger, soy sauce or tamari, sesame oil, rice vinegar, cornstarch, cooked brown rice or quinoa.

    - Instructions: Press tofu to remove excess water, then cut into cubes. Stir-fry tofu in a pan until golden brown. Add minced garlic and ginger, followed by mixed vegetables. Cook until vegetables are tender-crisp. In a bowl, mix soy sauce or tamari, sesame oil, rice vinegar, and cornstarch to make a sauce. Pour the sauce over the tofu and vegetables, and stir until thickened. Serve over cooked brown rice or quinoa.

2. Spaghetti with Vegan Marinara Sauce:

    - Ingredients: Whole grain spaghetti, marinara sauce (canned or homemade), garlic, onion, bell peppers, mushrooms, zucchini, fresh basil, nutritional yeast (optional).

    - Instructions: Cook whole grain spaghetti according to package instructions. In a separate pan, sauté minced garlic, diced onion, sliced bell peppers, sliced mushrooms, and diced zucchini until softened. Add marinara sauce and simmer until heated through. Serve marinara sauce over cooked spaghetti, garnished with fresh basil and nutritional yeast, if desired.

Snacks:

1. Hummus and Veggie Sticks:

    - Ingredients: Homemade or store-bought hummus, carrot sticks, cucumber slices, bell pepper strips, cherry tomatoes, celery sticks.

    - Instructions: Serve hummus with an assortment of fresh vegetable sticks for dipping. Enjoy as a nutritious and satisfying snack or appetizer.

2. Trail Mix:

    - Ingredients: Raw almonds, cashews, walnuts, pumpkin seeds, sunflower seeds, dried cranberries, dried apricots, dark chocolate chips.

    - Instructions: Mix together raw nuts, seeds, and dried fruits in a bowl. Store in an airtight container for a convenient and portable snack on the go.

These plant-based recipes are flavorful, satisfying, and packed with nutrients, making them perfect for anyone looking to incorporate more plant-based foods into their diet.

Overcoming Common Challenges

While switching to a plant-based diet has many advantages, there are drawbacks as well. The following are some typical obstacles that plant-based eating could run into, along with solutions:

1.Social Pressure: Eating plant-based can be difficult at times when you're among friends or at family get-togethers where the main course is usually meat or dairy. To deal with peer pressure, be mindful of your dietary choices and speak out about them. You might also offer to bring a plant-based dish to share or recommend vegan places.

2.Nutritional Adequacy: On a plant-based diet, making sure you obtain all the vital nutrients your body needs involves careful planning and close attention to detail. Focus on eating a range of full, nutrient-dense foods from all food categories to allay worries about nutritional sufficiency. You can also think about adding supplements or fortified foods as needed. For individualized advice and support, speak with a registered dietitian or other healthcare provider.

3.Cooking Skills: Those who are used to making meat-based meals may need to pick up new cooking methods and recipes while switching to a plant-based diet. Take culinary classes, watch online tutorials, try out easy plant-based dishes, and don't be afraid to experiment with flavors and ingredients to gain confidence in the kitchen.

4.Cravings and Taste Preferences: When switching to a plant-based diet, cravings for comfort foods and flavors, including cheese, meat, and processed snacks, may appear. Explore plant-based substitutes and alternatives, play around with different flavors and spices, and concentrate on integrating complete, minimally processed meals that are delicious and nutritious in order to satiate cravings and accommodate taste preferences.

5. Convenience and Accessibility: When eating out or traveling, it might be difficult to find plant-based options, particularly in places where fresh vegetables and vegetarian-friendly eateries are scarce. Plan ahead to research restaurant menus, prepare wholesome snacks and meals for travel, and stock up on pantry essentials and frozen foods for quick and simple meals at home in order to get beyond obstacles related to accessibility and convenience.

6. Family and Cultural Influences: Plant-based eating preferences can occasionally clash with family traditions, cultural conventions, and dietary habits, causing conflict or resistance from loved ones. To seek common ground by introducing plant-based recipes into shared meals, educate family members about the health and environmental benefits of a plant-based diet, address familial and cultural influences, and communicate in an open and courteous manner.

7. Budgetary Restrictions: Some people may be discouraged from implementing a plant-based diet due to the belief that it is costly or unaffordable. Prioritize inexpensive essentials like grains, legumes, fruits, and vegetables; purchase in bulk or during prime produce; check out your neighborhood farmers' markets or cheap grocery stores; and think about cultivating your own herbs or veggies at home to make a plant-based diet more affordable.

8. Time constraints: It might be difficult to prioritize meal planning, grocery shopping, and cooking due to demanding schedules and lifestyles. Invest in time-saving kitchen appliances and gadgets, use meal delivery services or plant-based meal kits, batch cook and

freeze meals in advance, and simplify recipes with few ingredients and cooking processes to save time and expedite meal preparation.

You may effectively overcome difficulties and make the switch to a plant-based diet that is in line with your ethical, environmental, and health beliefs by addressing these typical challenges with proactive techniques and a positive mentality.

Success Stories of People Who Eat Only Plants

Adopting a plant-based diet has helped many people achieve personal success and see miraculous health gains. Here are a few motivational tales of plant-based eaters' success:

1.Enhanced Health Markers: Many people who switched to a plant-based diet have noted notable changes in their health markers, such as decreased inflammation, better blood sugar regulation, lower cholesterol, and weight loss. Through the emphasis on nutrient-dense plant foods and the reduction or avoidance of animal products, they have improved their general health and wellbeing.

2.Weight Loss and Body Transformation: Because plant-based diets emphasize complete, minimally processed foods and increased fiber intake, they are frequently linked to benefits in body composition and weight loss. Adopting a plant-based diet has helped many people effectively lose extra weight, acquire lean muscle mass, increase their energy levels, and enhance their physical abilities.

3.Enhanced Athletic Performance: Plant-based diets have been shown to improve both athletic performance and recuperation for fitness enthusiasts and athletes. They have increased their power, stamina, endurance, and post-exercise recovery times by feeding their bodies with nutrient-dense plant meals. It has been demonstrated that plant-based diets enhance overall athletic excellence and support peak sports performance.

4.Chronic Illness Reversal: By adopting a plant-based diet and lifestyle, some people have been able to effectively reverse or manage chronic illnesses such type 2 diabetes, hypertension, cardiovascular disease, and autoimmune disorders. A whole-food, plant-based diet high in fruits, vegetables, whole grains, and legumes has significantly improved their quality of life and overall health.

5.Impact on the Environment and Ethics: A lot of people who consume plant-based foods do so because they want to make sure that their food choices support social justice, sustainability, and animal welfare. They are lessening their ecological footprint, protecting natural resources, and advancing a more just and humane food system by cutting back on or giving up their consumption of animal products.

These triumphs demonstrate the transforming potential of a plant-based diet in fostering energy, health, and overall well-being for people, communities, and the environment. You can start your own path to the best possible health, fulfillment, and happiness by adopting a plant-based diet and lifestyle.

In conclusion, there are many advantages to a plant-based diet for the environment, animal welfare, and human health. You may use the power of plants to nourish your body, mind, and spirit by putting an emphasis on nutrient-rich plant foods, incorporating a range of protein sources, making balanced meals, tasting delectable plant-based dishes, overcoming common obstacles, and finding inspiration from success stories. A plant-based diet can help you grow and flourish in many facets of your life, whether your goals are to decrease your environmental footprint, enhance your health, or match your eating habits with your principles.

CHAPTER EIGHT

DETOXIFICATION: SYSTEM PURIFICATION

The process of removing toxins and dangerous substances from the body in order to support general health, vitality, and well-being is known as detoxification, or detox. The significance of detoxification in healing, natural detox foods and beverages, secure and efficient detox techniques, sample detox plans and timetables, recipes for detoxifying meals and smoothies, supporting detox with lifestyle adjustments, and tracking your detox progress are all covered in this extensive book.

The Role of Detoxification in the Healing Process

We are exposed to many different kinds of toxins and pollutants in the modern world, such as chemicals found in household products, processed foods, pesticides, heavy metals, air and water pollution, and stress. These poisons can build up in the body over time and have a role in immune system malfunction, oxidative stress, inflammation, and chronic illness.

Supporting the body's natural detoxification processes and removing accumulated toxins from the body are two important functions of detoxification. In addition to promoting optimal health and recovery, aiding detoxification can lessen the strain on your eliminatory organs, including the liver, kidneys, lungs, skin, and lymphatic system.

Among the main advantages of detoxification are:

1.Better Digestive Health: Through encouraging regularity, eliminating waste and pollutants from the gastrointestinal tract, and improving nutrient absorption, detoxification improves digestive health. Detoxification can help reduce the symptoms of bloating, gas, constipation, and indigestion by promoting proper digestion and evacuation.

2.Enhanced Immune Function: To detect and get rid of infections, poisons, and foreign invaders, a healthy immune system needs to undergo appropriate detoxification. You can boost immunity and lower your chance of infections, allergies, and autoimmune diseases by encouraging detoxification.

3.Enhanced Vitality and Energy: Detoxification aids in the removal of built-up toxins that may hinder cellular processes and the generation of energy. You can increase general vitality and well-being, increase mental clarity, and increase energy levels by aiding in detoxification.

4.Weight management: Toxins that are deposited in adipose tissue can disrupt hormone balance and metabolism, leading to obesity and weight gain. You can encourage weight reduction, enhance metabolic efficiency, and expel stored toxins from fat cells by aiding in detoxification.

5.Clearer Skin: Skin conditions like acne, eczema, psoriasis, and poor complexion can be caused by toxins and impurities in the body. You can encourage a radiant complexion, lessen the visibility of skin flaws, and cleanse the skin from the inside out by aiding in detoxification.

6.Decreased Inflammation: A frequent underlying cause of many chronic diseases, such as diabetes, cancer, heart disease, and autoimmune disorders, is chronic inflammation. Supporting detoxification can help lower the body's inflammatory response, promote tissue regeneration and repair, and lessen the chance of developing chronic illnesses.

7.Balanced Hormones: Toxins and substances that disturb the endocrine system can tamper with hormone levels, causing irregular menstruation, infertility, and other reproductive problems. You can assist in maintaining reproductive health, promoting hormonal balance, and controlling hormone production and metabolism by assisting with detoxification.

Natural Remedy Foods and Beverages

Including nutrient-rich foods and beverages that assist the body's natural detoxification processes is one of the best methods to promote detoxification. You should incorporate the following natural detox foods and beverages into your diet:

1.Leafy Greens: Packed with chlorophyll, antioxidants, vitamins, and minerals, leafy greens including kale, spinach, Swiss chard, collard greens, and arugula help with cellular regeneration and liver cleansing. For optimal detoxification, incorporate a range of leafy greens into salads, smoothies, stir-fries, and juices.

2.Cruciferous Vegetables: Glucosinolates are substances found in cruciferous vegetables, like broccoli, Brussels sprouts, cabbage, cauliflower, and kale. These compounds help the liver detoxify and improve the body's capacity to get rid of toxins and carcinogens. Savor cruciferous veggies raw in salads and slaws, or cook them in a sauté, roast, or steam method.

3.Citrus Fruits: Packed with vitamin C, a potent antioxidant that aids in liver detoxification and strengthens the immune system, citrus fruits including lemons, limes, oranges, and grapefruits are abundant in this vitamin. Have a glass of warm lemon water to start your day, or infuse salads, marinades, and sauces with fresh citrus juice.

4.Berries: Packed with fiber, antioxidants, and phytonutrients, berries like strawberries, blueberries, raspberries, and blackberries aid in cellular detoxification and provide protection against oxidative stress. Berries can be added to smoothies, eaten as a snack when fresh or frozen, or added to oatmeal and yogurt for a healthy breakfast.

5.Fresh Herbs: Aside from their inherent cleansing qualities, fresh herbs like cilantro, parsley, dill, mint, and basil can also assist support kidney and liver function. Chopped herbs can be used as a garnish for your favorite recipes or added to salads, soups, sauces, and marinades.

6.Garlic and Onions: Packed with sulfur compounds, garlic and onions help the liver detoxify and improve the body's ability to get rid of heavy metals and toxins. Add onions and garlic to soups, stews, and other dishes by sautéing them with vegetables or using them as a base for marinades and sauces.

7.Strong anti-inflammatory spices like ginger and turmeric help liver cleansing, lower inflammation, and enhance general health and wellbeing. For extra taste and detoxifying effects, add fresh or powdered ginger and turmeric to drinks, smoothies, stir-fries, and curries.

8.Green Tea: Rich in catechins, an antioxidant class that supports liver function, accelerates fat metabolism, and improves detoxification, green tea has several health benefits. Drink green tea to rejuvenate yourself or add matcha powder to smoothies, lattes, and desserts to boost antioxidant content even further.

9.Herbs that are known to be naturally detoxifying include dandelion root, milk thistle, burdock root, and nettle leaf. These characteristics assist kidney and liver function, encourage bile movement, and improve the removal of toxins from the body. To aid in your detoxification efforts, take pleasure in these cleansing herbs as teas, tinctures, or supplements.

10.Water: Maintaining hydration is crucial for aiding in the body's detoxification and removal of pollutants. To maintain kidney function, encourage cellular hydration, and aid in the removal of waste products, drink lots of water throughout the day. For added taste and detoxifying effects, cut up fresh lemon or cucumber and add them to water.

You can assist your body's natural detoxification processes, improve general health, and feel better about yourself by including these natural detox foods and beverages in your diet.

Safe and Practical Detox Techniques

Detoxification has many health advantages, but in order to minimize dangers and consequences, it must be approached cautiously and correctly. Consider the following safe and efficient detoxification techniques:

1.Whole Foods Detox: To assist in the body's natural detoxification process, concentrate on eating a diet high in fruits, vegetables, whole grains, legumes, nuts, and seeds. Steer clear of processed meals, refined sugars, artificial chemicals, and unhealthy fats as these can all lead to inflammation and the buildup of toxins.

2.Hydration: To help with detoxification and hydration, sip herbal teas and lots of water throughout the day. Water stimulates renal function, encourages cellular hydration, and aids in the removal of toxins from the body. Drink as much water as possible throughout the day—at least 8–10 glasses—and think about flavoring your water with fresh lemon, cucumber, or mint for added health advantages.

3.Limit Toxin Exposure: Reduce the amount of environmental toxins you come into contact with by eating as much organic food as you can, avoiding packaged and processed foods that contain artificial additives and preservatives, using natural, non-toxic household cleaners and personal care products, filtering your tap water, and utilizing fewer plastics and other disposable items.

4.Promote Liver Health: The liver is the body's main organ for detoxification; it breaks down and gets rid of poisons. You may promote the health of your liver by eating a diet high in nutrients, avoiding alcohol, using supplements and medications sparingly, and including foods and herbs that are good for the liver, such milk thistle, dandelion root, artichokes, beets, and carrots.

5. Encourage Digestive Health: Eat a diet high in fiber, drink plenty of water, and include foods high in probiotics, including kimchi, sauerkraut, kefir, and yogurt, in your meals to help detoxification. Probiotics assist immune system health and gut health, while fiber aids in the binding of toxins in the gut and encourages regular bowel movements.

6. Reduce Your Stress: Prolonged stress can hinder the body's ability to detoxify and increase the buildup of toxins. Utilize methods of reducing stress, such as yoga, tai chi, deep breathing, meditation, and time spent in nature, to enhance general wellbeing, induce relaxation, and lower stress hormones.

7. Exercise Frequently: By encouraging circulation, lymphatic drainage, and sweating, which aids in the removal of toxins through the skin, physical exercise aids in detoxification. To help detoxification and general health, try to get regular exercise, such as walking, jogging, cycling, swimming, or yoga.

8. Sauna Therapy: By causing perspiration and removing toxins through the skin, sauna therapy can aid in the detoxification process. If you want to enhance detoxification, ease muscle tension, and enhance general wellbeing, think about adding frequent sauna sessions to your health regimen. To avoid dehydration, make sure you drink enough of water before to, during, and after sauna sessions.

9. Intermittent Fasting: To assist detoxification, enhance metabolic health, and encourage cellular repair and regeneration, intermittent

fasting alternates between eating and fasting intervals. To enhance detoxification and general health, think about including intermittent fasting techniques like time-restricted eating, fasting on alternate days, or periodic fasting into your daily regimen.

10. Speak with a trained Healthcare Professional: It's crucial to get advice from a trained healthcare provider, such as a registered dietitian, nutritionist, or functional medicine practitioner, before beginning any detox program or making big dietary or lifestyle changes. They can assist in determining the specific health requirements you have, make tailored advice, and guarantee that the detoxification techniques you select are secure and suitable for you.

You may increase general health, heighten your sense of well-being, and assist your body's natural detoxification processes by implementing these safe and efficient detox procedures into daily regimen.

Sample Detox Plans and Schedules

Detox plans and schedules can vary depending on individual health goals, preferences, and needs. Here are some sample detox plans and schedules to consider:

3-Day Whole Foods Detox Plan:

Day 1:

- Upon Waking: Drink a glass of warm lemon water to support hydration and detoxification.

- Breakfast: Green smoothie made with leafy greens, cucumber, celery, parsley, lemon juice, and coconut water.

- Mid-Morning Snack: Fresh berries such as strawberries, blueberries, or raspberries.

- Lunch: Mixed green salad with spinach, arugula, cherry tomatoes, cucumber, avocado, and pumpkin seeds, dressed with olive oil and lemon juice.

- Afternoon Snack: Raw veggies such as carrot sticks, celery, and bell pepper strips with hummus.

- Dinner: Grilled salmon or tofu with steamed broccoli, roasted sweet potatoes, and sautéed kale with garlic.

Day 2:

- Upon Waking: Drink a glass of warm lemon water.

- Breakfast: Overnight oats made with rolled oats, almond milk, chia seeds, sliced banana, and cinnamon.

- Mid-Morning Snack: Sliced apple with almond butter.

- Lunch: Quinoa salad with mixed vegetables, chickpeas, diced bell pepper, cucumber, parsley, and lemon-tahini dressing.

- Afternoon Snack: Raw nuts such as almonds, walnuts, or cashews.

- Dinner: Stir-fried tempeh or tofu with mixed veggies (bell peppers, broccoli, snap peas) in a ginger-garlic sauce served over brown rice.

Day 3:

- Upon Waking: Drink a glass of warm lemon water.
- Breakfast: Green smoothie bowl topped with sliced kiwi, berries, coconut flakes, and hemp seeds.
- Mid-Morning Snack: Celery sticks with almond butter and raisins (ants on a log).
- Lunch: Lentil soup with carrots, celery, onions, garlic, tomatoes, spinach, and vegetable broth.
- Afternoon Snack: Homemade trail mix with raw nuts, seeds, and dried fruits.
- Dinner: Baked cod or roasted portobello mushrooms with quinoa pilaf and steamed asparagus.

7-Day Plant-Based Detox Plan:

Day 1:

- Upon Waking: Drink a glass of warm lemon water.
- Breakfast: Green smoothie with kale, spinach, banana, pineapple, ginger, and coconut water.
- Mid-Morning Snack: Fresh fruit salad with mixed berries, melon, and grapes.
- Lunch: Chickpea and vegetable stir-fry with broccoli, bell peppers, snap peas, carrots, garlic, and ginger served over brown rice.
- Afternoon Snack: Raw veggies with guacamole or salsa.

- Dinner: Stuffed bell peppers with quinoa, black beans, corn, diced tomatoes, onions, and spices, served with a side salad.

Day 2:

- Upon Waking: Drink a glass of warm lemon water.
- Breakfast: Overnight chia pudding made with almond milk, chia seeds, vanilla extract, and mixed berries.
- Mid-Morning Snack: Handful of raw almonds or cashews.
- Lunch: Lentil and vegetable soup with carrots, celery, onions, garlic, tomatoes, kale, and vegetable broth.
- Afternoon Snack: Sliced cucumber with hummus or tahini.
- Dinner: Baked tofu or tempeh with roasted Brussels sprouts, sweet potatoes, and a kale salad with lemon-tahini dressing.

Day 3:

- Upon Waking: Drink a glass of warm lemon water.
- Breakfast: Acai bowl topped with granola, sliced banana, shredded coconut, and goji berries.
- Mid-Morning Snack: Sliced apple with almond butter.
- Lunch: Quinoa salad with mixed greens, cherry tomatoes, cucumber, avocado, pumpkin seeds, and balsamic vinaigrette.
- Afternoon Snack: Raw veggies with guacamole or salsa.

- Dinner: Vegetable stir-fry with tofu or tempeh, bell peppers, broccoli, snap peas, carrots, garlic, and ginger, served over brown rice or quinoa.

Day 4:

- Upon Waking: Drink a glass of warm lemon water.
- Breakfast: Smoothie bowl with mixed berries, spinach, banana, almond milk, and a scoop of plant-based protein powder, topped with granola and sliced kiwi.
- Mid-Morning Snack: Raw nuts such as walnuts or almonds.
- Lunch: Mediterranean quinoa salad with diced cucumber, cherry tomatoes, red onion, Kalamata olives, fresh parsley, lemon juice, and olive oil.
- Afternoon Snack: Carrot and celery sticks with hummus.
- Dinner: Roasted vegetable Buddha bowl with roasted sweet potatoes, Brussels sprouts, cauliflower, chickpeas, and tahini dressing.

Day 5:

- Upon Waking: Drink a glass of warm lemon water.
- Breakfast: Overnight oats with rolled oats, almond milk, chia seeds, maple syrup, and sliced strawberries.
- Mid-Morning Snack: Fresh fruit such as grapes or orange slices.

- Lunch: Black bean and corn salad with diced bell pepper, red onion, cilantro, lime juice, and avocado.
- Afternoon Snack: Rice cakes with almond butter and sliced banana.
- Dinner: Lentil and vegetable curry with coconut milk, diced tomatoes, onion, garlic, ginger, curry powder, and spinach, served with brown rice.

Day 6:

- Upon Waking: Drink a glass of warm lemon water.
- Breakfast: Green smoothie with kale, spinach, mango, pineapple, coconut water, and a scoop of spirulina or chlorella powder.
- Mid-Morning Snack: Trail mix with raw nuts, seeds, and dried fruit.
- Lunch: Spinach and avocado salad with sliced strawberries, toasted almonds, red onion, and balsamic vinaigrette.
- Afternoon Snack: Sliced cucumber with hummus or guacamole.
- Dinner: Grilled portobello mushrooms with quinoa pilaf and steamed broccolini.

Day 7:

- Upon Waking: Drink a glass of warm lemon water.
- Breakfast: Acai smoothie bowl topped with granola, sliced banana, shredded coconut, and goji berries.

- Mid-Morning Snack: Fresh fruit salad with mixed berries, melon, and grapes.
- Lunch: Chickpea and vegetable stir-fry with broccoli, bell peppers, snap peas, carrots, garlic, and ginger served over brown rice.
- Afternoon Snack: Raw veggies with hummus or tahini.
- Dinner: Baked tofu or tempeh with roasted Brussels sprouts, sweet potatoes, and a kale salad with lemon-tahini dressing.

These sample detox plans provide a framework for incorporating nutrient-rich plant-based foods into your diet to support detoxification, promote overall health, and enhance your sense of well-being. Feel free to modify and customize these plans based on your individual preferences, dietary restrictions, and health goals.

Recipes for Detoxifying Meals and Smoothies

Here are some delicious and nutritious recipes for detoxifying meals and smoothies to support your detoxification efforts:

Detoxifying Meals:

1. Green Detox Salad:

- Ingredients:
    - 4 cups mixed greens (spinach, kale, arugula)
    - 1 cucumber, sliced

- 1 cup cherry tomatoes, halved
- 1 avocado, diced
- 1/4 cup pumpkin seeds
- 1/4 cup fresh cilantro, chopped
- Lemon-Tahini Dressing:
  - 2 tablespoons tahini
  - 2 tablespoons lemon juice
  - 1 tablespoon olive oil
  - 1 clove garlic, minced
  - Salt and pepper to taste
- Instructions:

1. In a large bowl, combine mixed greens, sliced cucumber, cherry tomatoes, diced avocado, pumpkin seeds, and chopped cilantro.

2. In a small bowl, whisk together tahini, lemon juice, olive oil, minced garlic, salt, and pepper until smooth and creamy.

3. Drizzle the lemon-tahini dressing over the salad and toss gently to coat.

4. Serve immediately and enjoy!

2. Detoxifying Vegetable Stir-Fry:
- Ingredients:

- 1 tablespoon coconut oil
- 1 block tofu or tempeh, cubed
- 2 cups mixed vegetables (bell peppers, broccoli, snap peas, carrots)
- 2 cloves garlic, minced
- 1 tablespoon grated ginger
- 2 tablespoons tamari or soy sauce
- 1 tablespoon rice vinegar
- 1 teaspoon maple syrup
- Cooked brown rice or quinoa, for serving
- Instructions:

1. Heat coconut oil in a large skillet or wok over medium heat. Add cubed tofu or tempeh and cook until golden brown on all sides, about 5-7 minutes. Remove from skillet and set aside.

2. In the same skillet, add mixed vegetables, minced garlic, and grated ginger. Stir-fry for 3-5 minutes until vegetables are tender-crisp.

3. In a small bowl, whisk together tamari or soy sauce, rice vinegar, and maple syrup. Pour the sauce over the vegetables and return the tofu or tempeh to the skillet. Stir-fry for an additional 2-3 minutes until heated through.

4. Serve the vegetable stir-fry over cooked brown rice or quinoa and enjoy!

3. Detoxifying Lentil Soup:

- Ingredients:
- 1 tablespoon olive oil
- 1 onion, diced
- 2 carrots, diced
- 2 celery stalks, diced
- 3 cloves garlic, minced
- 1 teaspoon ground cumin
- 1 teaspoon ground turmeric
- 1/2 teaspoon ground coriander
- 1 cup dried green lentils, rinsed and drained
- 4 cups vegetable broth
- 1 can (14 oz) diced tomatoes
- 2 cups chopped kale or spinach
- Salt and pepper to taste
- Instructions:

1. Heat olive oil in a large pot over medium heat. Add diced onion, carrots, and celery, and sauté for 5-7 minutes until vegetables are softened.

2. Add minced garlic, ground cumin, ground turmeric, and ground coriander, and sauté for an additional 1-2 minutes until fragrant.

3. Add dried green lentils, vegetable broth, and diced tomatoes to the pot. Bring to a boil, then reduce heat and simmer for 20-25 minutes until lentils are tender. 4. Stir in chopped kale or spinach and cook for an additional 5 minutes until greens are wilted. 5. Season with salt and pepper to taste. 6. Serve hot and enjoy this nourishing and detoxifying lentil soup!

Detoxifying Smoothies:

1. Green Detox Smoothie:
- Ingredients:
- 1 cup spinach
- 1/2 cup kale
- 1/2 cucumber, peeled and chopped
- 1/2 green apple, cored and chopped
- 1/2 lemon, juiced
- 1 tablespoon fresh ginger, grated
- 1 tablespoon chia seeds
- 1 cup coconut water or almond milk
- Ice cubes (optional)
- Instructions:

1. Place spinach, kale, cucumber, green apple, lemon juice, grated ginger, chia seeds, and coconut water or almond milk in a blender.

2. Blend on high speed until smooth and creamy.

3. Add ice cubes if desired and blend again until well combined.

4. Pour into glasses and enjoy this refreshing and detoxifying green smoothie!

   2. Berry Detox Smoothie:
   - Ingredients:
   - 1 cup mixed berries (strawberries, blueberries, raspberries)
   - 1/2 banana, peeled
   - 1 tablespoon ground flaxseeds
   - 1 tablespoon hemp seeds
   - 1 tablespoon fresh lemon juice
   - 1 cup almond milk or coconut water
   - Ice cubes (optional)
   - Instructions:

1. Combine mixed berries, banana, ground flaxseeds, hemp seeds, fresh lemon juice, and almond milk or coconut water in a blender.

2. Blend on high speed until smooth and creamy.

3. Add ice cubes if desired and blend again until well combined.

4. Pour into glasses and enjoy this delicious and antioxidant-rich berry smoothie!

3. Tropical Detox Smoothie:

- Ingredients:
- 1/2 cup pineapple chunks
- 1/2 cup mango chunks
- 1/2 banana, peeled
- 1 tablespoon shredded coconut
- 1 tablespoon fresh lime juice
- 1 tablespoon chia seeds
- 1 cup coconut water or almond milk
- Ice cubes (optional)
- Instructions:

1. Place pineapple chunks, mango chunks, banana, shredded coconut, fresh lime juice, chia seeds, and coconut water or almond milk in a blender.

2. Blend on high speed until smooth and creamy.

3. Add ice cubes if desired and blend again until well combined.

4.   Pour into glasses and enjoy this tropical and refreshing detox smoothie!

These detoxifying meals and smoothies are packed with nutrient-rich ingredients that support the body's natural detoxification processes, promote overall health, and enhance your sense of well-being. Incorporate these recipes into your detox plan to nourish your body and support your detoxification journey.

Supporting Detox with Lifestyle Changes

Apart from dietary adjustments, lifestyle improvements can bolster detoxification even more and improve your general health. Consider making the following lifestyle adjustments:

1.Stress Reduction: Prolonged stress can impede the body's detoxification processes and lead to a build-up of toxins. To encourage relaxation, lower stress hormones, and aid in detoxification, try stress-reduction methods including deep breathing, meditation, yoga, tai chi, and spending time in nature.

2.Frequent Exercise: Exercise aids in detoxification by enhancing lymphatic drainage, circulation, and sweating, all of which aid in the removal of toxins through the skin. To help detoxification and general health, try to get regular exercise, such as walking, jogging, cycling, swimming, or yoga.

3.Sufficient Sleep: Both detoxification and general health depend on getting enough good sleep. To promote hormone balance, immune system performance, and cellular repair and regeneration, aim for 7-9 hours of restorative sleep each night. To encourage sound sleep, establish a calming nighttime routine, abstain from coffee and gadgets before bed, and furnish your bedroom with comfy furnishings.

4. Drinking enough water is crucial to aiding in the body's detoxification and removal of pollutants. To maintain kidney function, encourage cellular hydration, and aid in the removal of waste products, drink lots of water throughout the day. For added taste and detoxification, squeeze in some fresh lemon, cucumber, or mint into your water.

5. Sauna Therapy: By causing perspiration and removing toxins through the skin, sauna therapy can aid in the detoxification process. If you want to enhance detoxification, ease muscle tension, and enhance general wellbeing, think about adding frequent sauna sessions to your health regimen. To avoid dehydration, make sure you drink enough of water before to, during, and after sauna sessions.

6. Eat with awareness: Make conscious eating choices by chewing food well, eating slowly, and observing your body's signals of hunger and fullness. Steer clear of distractions like screens and multitasking when eating, and chew your food slowly to improve digestion, vitamin absorption, and overall meal enjoyment.

7. Limit Your Consumption of Alcohol and Caffeine: These substances can tax the liver and impede the liver's detoxifying processes. Drink less alcohol and caffeine-containing drinks (coffee, tea, energy drinks), and go for healthy options like sparkling water, herbal teas, or water.

8. Environmental Detox: Reduce your exposure to environmental toxins by drinking tap water that has been filtered, avoiding

packaged and processed foods that contain artificial additives and preservatives, opting for organic foods whenever possible, and using natural, non-toxic household and personal care products.

You may further boost detoxification, improve general health, and elevate your sense of well-being by implementing these lifestyle modifications into your everyday routine.

Tracking the Progress of Your Detox

You may track your health improvements, pinpoint areas that need more optimization, and maintain motivation for your wellness journey by keeping track of your detox progress. Here are some methods to track the progress of your detox:

1.Maintain a Detox record: Begin keeping a record of your food consumption, water intake, physical activity, stress levels, sleep habits, and any symptoms or health changes. Keep a journal of your meals, snacks, and drinks, along with any sentiments or ideas you have about your detoxification journey. To keep yourself accountable and inspired, periodically reflect on your accomplishments, obstacles, and growth.

2.Monitor Physical Symptoms: Be mindful of any alterations in physical manifestations, including but not limited to energy levels, digestion, skin health, mood, and sleep quality. Keep an eye out for any changes in symptoms, such as higher energy, clearer skin, better digestion, happier mood, and more restful sleep; these could be signs that your detoxification efforts are working.

3.Measurements and Biomarkers: Before, during, and after your detox program, think about keeping track of objective measurements and biomarkers including weight, body composition, blood pressure, cholesterol levels, blood sugar levels, inflammatory indicators, and detoxification markers (such liver enzymes). Speak with a medical expert to understand your results and evaluate your development over time.

4.Evaluate your emotional health: detoxification involves not just physical but also mental and emotional cleansing. Take note of any improvements in your emotional health, such as lowered stress and anxiety, happier feelings, sharper mind, and increased ability to withstand stress. Throughout your detox journey, pay attention to your thoughts, feelings, and general sense of wellbeing. Celebrate any improvements or breakthroughs in your mental and emotional well-being.

5.Speak with a Qualified Healthcare Professional: For individualized advice and assistance during your detoxification process, it's crucial to speak with a certified dietitian, nutritionist, or functional medicine practitioner. They may assist in determining your unique health requirements, keeping an eye on your development, modifying your detox plan as necessary, and resolving any issues or difficulties that come up during the process.

6.Listen to Your Body: In the end, paying attention to your body's signals and cues is the most crucial way to track your detoxification progress. Consider the effects that various foods, beverages, pastimes, and lifestyle choices have on your physical, mental, and spiritual well-being. When making changes to improve your general health and well-being, follow your gut.

Through consistent monitoring of your detox process and awareness of your body's requirements, you may maximize your efforts towards detoxification, support general health, and improve your overall feeling of energy and wellbeing.

To sum up, detoxification is essential for maintaining health and wellbeing because it aids the body's natural mechanisms for getting rid of toxins and dangerous materials. You may boost detoxification, improve general health, and heighten your sense of vitality and well-being by implementing nutrient-rich meals and beverages, safe and effective detox procedures, lifestyle modifications, and progress monitoring in addition to other strategies. For individualized advice and assistance, never forget to speak with a healthcare provider. Additionally, pay attention to your body's signs and signals as you proceed through your detox. You can start a detoxification journey that nourishes your body, mind, and spirit and gives you the tools to live your healthiest and happiest life with commitment, awareness, and self-care.

CHAPTER NINE
BOOSTING YOUR IMMUNE SYSTEM ORGANICALLY

Your body uses the immune system as a line of defense against noxious pathogens, such as bacteria, viruses, and other germs, in addition to poisons and foreign objects. Sustaining general health and averting infections and diseases requires a strong immune system. Immune health is greatly influenced by a person's diet, exercise routine, stress reduction techniques, sleep patterns, and social support, in addition to hereditary variables. Here's how to naturally boost your immune system:

1. Anti-Immune Foods and Herbs

A diet high in nutrients is essential for maintaining general health and immune system function. A few foods and herbs include more vitamins, minerals, antioxidants, and phytochemicals than others, which makes them especially useful for strengthening immunity. Include the following foods and herbs in your diet to strengthen your immune system:

• Citrus Fruits: Vitamin C, a strong antioxidant that boosts the development of white blood cells, which aid in the fight against infections, is abundant in citrus fruits, including oranges, lemons, limes, and grapefruits.

• Berries: Rich in antioxidants such as vitamin C and polyphenols, berries such as strawberries, blueberries, raspberries, and blackberries fortify the immune system and guard against oxidative stress.

• Garlic: Allicin, a chemical found in garlic, has immune-stimulating and antibacterial qualities. Regular garlic consumption may boost immune function and lower the risk of infection.

• Ginger: Due to its anti-inflammatory and antioxidant qualities, ginger may boost immunity and lessen the intensity and protracted course of respiratory infections.

• Turmeric: The plant's primary ingredient, curcumin, has strong antioxidant and anti-inflammatory properties. Including turmeric in your diet may help control inflammatory and immunological reactions.

• Green leafy vegetables: High in vitamins, minerals, and antioxidants, these veggies promote healthy immune system function and general well-being. Examples of these veggies are collard greens, spinach, kale, and Swiss chard.

• Medicinal Mushrooms: A number of mushrooms, including cordyceps, shiitake, maitake, and reishi, include bioactive substances with immunomodulatory qualities that may improve immune function.

• Echinacea: This herb is frequently used to boost immune function and lessen the intensity and length of colds and the flu. It might strengthen the body's defenses against infections and encourage the activation of immune cells.

• Elderberry: Packed with vitamins and antioxidants, elderberries enhance immune system performance. It has been used traditionally to treat respiratory infections, the flu, and colds. It may also help lessen symptoms and shorten the course of disease.

To make sure you're obtaining the necessary nutrients to promote immune function, focus on eating a varied and balanced diet rich in fruits, vegetables, whole grains, lean meats, and healthy fats in addition to including these immune-boosting foods and herbs in your diet.

2. The Value of Frequent Exercise

Engaging in consistent physical activity is crucial for preserving immune system function in addition to cardiovascular health, strength, and endurance. Numerous positive impacts of exercise on the immune system have been demonstrated, including:

• Boosting Immune Surveillance: Physical activity promotes the body's circulation of white blood cells, antibodies, and other immune cells, which improves the body's ability to recognize and react to infections.

• Reducing Chronic Inflammation: Reducing chronic inflammation can boost the risk of developing chronic diseases and impede immune function. By influencing immunological responses and encouraging the release of anti-inflammatory cytokines, regular exercise helps lower inflammation.

• Enhancing Stress Response: Exercise is a natural way to lower stress hormone levels, such as cortisol, which, when persistently raised, can impair immune function.

• Enhancing Sleep Quality: Getting regular exercise helps lengthen and enhance sleep, which is crucial for immune system performance and general health.

Aim for two or more days of muscle-strengthening exercises per week in addition to at least 150 minutes of moderate-intensity aerobic activity or 75 minutes of vigorous-intensity aerobic exercise every week. Running, hiking, and high-intensity interval training (HIIT) are examples of vigorous-intensity exercises, whereas brisk walking, cycling, swimming, and dancing are examples of moderate-intensity aerobic exercise. Making exercise a regular part of your lifestyle and keeping yourself motivated can be achieved by incorporating a number of enjoyable activities.

3. Techniques for Stress Management

Long-term stress can negatively impact immune function and make a person more vulnerable to infections and diseases. Therefore, in order to maintain immunological health and general well-being, it is imperative that you include stress management practices into your daily routine. The following are some practical methods for reducing stress:

• Deep Breathing: Deep breathing techniques, such diaphragmatic breathing, can lower stress hormones, trigger the body's relaxation response, and encourage feelings of serenity and relaxation. Several times a day, or whenever you're feeling worried or agitated, spend a few minutes practicing deep breathing.

• Progressive Muscle Relaxation: To relieve stress and encourage relaxation, progressive muscle relaxation entails tensing and relaxing various bodily muscle groups. For a few seconds, tense a particular muscle group. Then, release the tension and relax, paying attention to the feeling of relaxation. Proceed to the tips of your toes and repeat this procedure for every muscle group.

- Mindfulness Meditation: This technique entails focusing on the here and now without passing judgment and letting go of ideas, emotions, and sensations as they arise. Frequent mindfulness meditation practice has been demonstrated to boost immunity and lessen stress, anxiety, and depression.

- Yoga: Yoga promotes relaxation, lowers stress levels, and improves general well-being by combining physical postures, breathwork, and meditation. Regular yoga practice can lower stress levels and strengthen the immune system while enhancing flexibility, strength, balance, and mental clarity.

- Tai Chi and Qigong: Tai Chi and Qigong are mind-body exercises that encourage energy flow, balance, and relaxation through slow, deliberate motions, deep breathing, and meditation. Research has demonstrated that these age-old methods can lower stress, elevate mood, and strengthen the immune system.

4. Practices of Mindfulness and Meditation

Techniques for mindfulness and meditation are effective ways to lower stress, encourage relaxation, and improve general wellbeing. By engaging in these activities, you can develop an awareness of the present moment that is characterized by acceptance, curiosity, and openness, which will help you become resilient and peaceful within. Consider the following mindfulness and meditation techniques:

- Breath Awareness: Just paying attention to your breathing's natural rhythm will help you focus on the here and now and de-stress. Spend a few seconds concentrating on how your breath feels entering and exiting your body. Pay attention to how your chest or abdomen rises and falls with each breath.

- Body Scan: This type of meditation is methodically focusing attention on various body parts, beginning at the top of the head and working your way down to the toes. With every breath, allow any tension or discomfort that you feel as you go through your body to soften and release.

- Loving-Kindness Meditation: This type of meditation focuses on developing positive thoughts and feelings for both yourself and other people. Start by reciting aloud affirmations like "May I be happy, may I be healthy, may I be safe, may I be at ease," initially to oneself and then progressively to family, friends, and all living things.

- Mindfulness in Daily Activities: By giving whatever you're doing in the present moment your whole attention, you can cultivate mindfulness in your daily activities. Try not to let thoughts of the past or the future divert you from the present moment as you eat, walk, wash dishes, or brush your teeth. Take in the sights, sounds, smells, and sensations that surround you, and relish the richness of every moment.

- Guided Meditations: You can practice mindfulness and meditation with the help of guided meditation apps or audio recordings. A vast array of subjects are covered in guided meditations, ranging from relaxation and stress relief to self-compassion and thankfulness. Regularly listening to guided meditations will help you develop your practice and become more attentive in your day-to-day activities.

5. Establishing a Sound Sleep Schedule

For the immune system to work properly, general health, and wellbeing, quality sleep is crucial. The body strengthens memories, renews and repairs tissues, and boosts immunity while we sleep.

Deficient sleep or inadequate sleep can exacerbate inflammation, damage the immune system, and negatively impact mood and cognitive abilities. Use these suggestions to establish a healthy sleep schedule that can maximize your sleep and boost your immune system:

• Regular Bedtime: Even on the weekends, stick to a regular sleep routine by going to bed and waking up at the same time each day. Maintaining consistency improves the quality of your sleep and aids your body's internal clock.

• Establish a Calm nighttime Routine: Establish a calming nighttime routine to let your body know when it's time to unwind and get ready for sleep. You can encourage relaxation and make the transition to sleep easier by engaging in activities like reading, having a warm bath, practicing relaxation techniques, or listening to relaxing music.

• Minimize Screen Time Before Bed: Using devices like TVs, laptops, tablets, and cellphones right before bed can interfere with melatonin production, a hormone that controls sleep-wake cycles, and disturb sleep patterns. Reduce the amount of time spent on screens an hour or more before bed, and think about utilizing blue light filters or lowering the brightness of screens at night.

• Establish a Comfortable Sleep Environment: Keep your bedroom quiet, dark, and cold to promote restful sleep. Invest in cozy pillows and mattresses, block out light with blackout curtains or eye masks, and muffle distracting noises with earplugs or white noise devices.

• Limit Alcohol and Caffeine: These substances can disturb sleep patterns and impair the quality of sleep. Alcohol should be avoided close to bedtime as it can interfere with REM sleep and cause nightly awakenings. Limit your use of caffeinated beverages such as coffee, tea, and soda, especially in the afternoon and evening.

• **Practice Relaxation Techniques:** To calm the body and mind and encourage sound sleep, practice relaxation techniques like progressive muscle relaxation, deep breathing, or mindfulness meditation before bed.

You may improve immune system function, maximize the quality of your sleep, and improve your general health and well-being by making sleep a priority and developing a good sleep schedule.

6. Creating a Helpful Environment

Mental, emotional, and physical well-being depend on social ties and a nurturing atmosphere. Strong social support has been associated with superior health outcomes, a stronger immune system, and lower levels of stress. The following are some strategies for creating a nurturing atmosphere and developing deep relationships:

• **Establish a Connection with Loved Ones:** Make time for friends, family, and loved ones that encourage and support you. Have deep discussions, exchange personal stories, and provide one another with moral support and encouragement.

• **Join Communities:** Assemble groups in your neighborhood that have similar interests or pastimes. Take part in classes, events, or group activities where you can network with like-minded people and form friendships.

• **Seek Professional Support:** Consult a therapist, counselor, or mental health professional for assistance if you're experiencing stress, anxiety, or other mental health issues. Speaking with a qualified expert can offer insightful advice, coping mechanisms, and support during trying times.

• Volunteer: To give back to the community and support causes you care about, become engaged in volunteer work or community service projects. Volunteering helps you meet people who share your interests and values and gives you a sense of fulfillment and purpose.

• Practice Gratitude: Develop an attitude of thankfulness by emphasizing the good things in your life and expressing your gratitude to the people and things that bring you joy. Write thank-you notes, keep a gratitude notebook, or just spend a time every day to consider and appreciate your benefits.

You may improve your well-being, boost immunity, and fortify your resilience by creating a loving atmosphere and fostering meaningful relationships with others.

To sum up, maintaining immunological function is critical for general wellbeing and for resiliency against diseases and infections. You can naturally strengthen your immune system and improve your capacity to thrive in all facets of life by including immune-boosting foods and herbs in your diet, making regular exercise a priority, practicing stress management techniques, developing mindfulness and meditation practices, developing a healthy sleep schedule, and creating a supportive environment. Keep in mind that over time, minor, regular adjustments to lifestyle choices can have a big influence on immune system performance and general health. Make self-care a priority, pay attention to what your body needs, and ask for help from loved ones and medical professionals when you need it. You can maintain and improve your health and wellbeing for years to come by using a comprehensive strategy for immune support.

www.ingramcontent.com/pod-product-compliance
Lightning Source LLC
Chambersburg PA
CBHW051105261224
19523CB00012B/143